Health Reference Series Online **Activation Code:**

ja4769

To activate this title in your online database, go to "Settings" and enter the above Activation Code into the appropriate field.

To set up your online *Health Reference Series* database for the first time, go to www.online.omnigraphics.com/registration

Questions? Call (800) 234-1340, email help@omnigraphics.com or go to www.omnigraphics.com/health-reference-online

ANXIETY DISORDERS
SOURCEBOOK

SECOND EDITION

Health Reference Series

ANXIETY DISORDERS
SOURCEBOOK

SECOND EDITION

Basic Consumer Health Information about Prevalence, Risk Factors, Types, Diagnosis, and Treatment of Anxiety Disorders

Along with Facts about Comorbidities of Anxiety Disorders, Managing Symptoms of Anxiety, Financial Assistance and Support, and Resources for Additional Help and Information

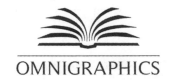

OMNIGRAPHICS

615 Griswold St., Ste. 520, Detroit, MI 48226

Library of Congress Cataloging-in-Publication Data

Names: Hayes, Kevin (Editor of health information), editor.

Title: Anxiety disorders sourcebook / edited by Kevin Hayes, basic consumer health Information about mental-health disorders and associated myths and facts, types of anxiety disorders, including general anxiety disorder, obsessive-compulsive disorder, posttraumatic stress disorder, panic disorder, social anxiety disorder, specific phobia, separation anxiety, illness anxiety disorder, somatic symptom disorder, and more along with information about causes, risk factors, treatment options, including medication, psychotherapy, and complementary and alternative medications, financial assistance, tips for caregivers, a glossary of related terms, and a directory of resources for more information.

Description: Second edition. | Detroit, MI: Omnigraphics, [2020] | Series: Health reference series | Includes bibliographical references and index. | Summary: "Provides consumer health information about the ways people encounter anxiety and its various types, including general anxiety disorder, obsessive-compulsive disorder, posttraumatic stress disorder (PTSD), and panic disorder. Includes glossary, index, and other resources"-- Provided by publisher.

Identifiers: LCCN 2020025293 (print) | LCCN 2020025294 (ebook) | ISBN 9780780818187 (library binding) | ISBN 9780780818194 (ebook)

Subjects: LCSH: Anxiety disorders--Popular works.

Classification: LCC RC531.A6137 2020 (print) | LCC RC531 (ebook) | DDC 616.85/22--dc23

LC record available at https://lccn.loc.gov/2020025293
LC ebook record available at https://lccn.loc.gov/2020025294

Table of Contents

Part 4. Psychiatric Comorbidities in Anxiety Disorder

Part 8. Additional Help and Information

Preface

ABOUT THIS BOOK

Concerns over finances, work, family, and the future are common sources of anxiety. In many cases individuals cope with such stressors and lead a healthy life. However, for others, worry becomes uncontrollable, taking a profound physical and mental toll. Prolonged anxiety can also lead to severe conditions such as depression, heart disease, and diabetes, and may also make an individual more vulnerable to substance abuse.

Anxiety Disorders Sourcebook, Second Edition provides an overview of anxiety disorders and highlights its potential risk factors. It discusses anxiety disorders in specific populations such as children, teens, pregnant women, older adults, and the LGBTQ community. It offers facts about the most common types of anxiety disorders including generalized anxiety disorder (GAD), separation anxiety disorder, specific phobias, social anxiety disorder (SAD), selective mutism, etc. Diagnosis and treatment of anxiety disorders are discussed in detail. The book provides information about psychiatric comorbidities in anxiety disorder such as attention deficit hyperactivity disorder (ADHD), bipolar disorder, borderline personality disorder (BPD), depression, eating disorders, and so on. It explains how individuals can manage and cope with the symptoms of anxiety and lead productive lives. It talks about financial assistance and support available for people with mental-health problems. Information about several anxiety-related research activities are also provided. The book concludes with a glossary of terms related to anxiety disorders and directories of mental-health resources and organizations for people with anxiety disorders and other mental concerns.

HOW TO USE THIS BOOK

This book is divided into parts and chapters. Parts focus on broad areas of interest. Chapters are devoted to single topics within a part.

Part 1: Introduction to Mental-Health and Anxiety Disorders begins with an overview of mental health and mental illness. It dispels common myths and provides facts about mental health. It discusses anxiety disorders in general and highlights the potential risk factors for anxiety disorders. It provides statistical information on anxiety disorders and its incidence in specific populations.

Part 2: Types of Anxiety Disorders gives an overview of the most common types of anxiety disorders including generalized anxiety disorder (GAD), separation anxiety disorder, specific phobias, social anxiety disorder (SAD), selective mutism, panic disorders, agoraphobia, and substance- or medication-induced anxiety disorder.

Part 3: General Principles of Diagnosis and Treatment provides information about diagnosis of anxiety disorders. Therapies for alleviating anxiety disorders such as psychotherapy, cognitive-behavioral therapy (CBT), and medications have been included. Complementary health approaches including relaxation techniques, yoga, tai chi, qi gong, massage therapy, art and play therapy, etc. are also discussed. It highlights the importance of support groups and integrating behavioral health services into primary care.

Part 4: Psychiatric Comorbidities in Anxiety Disorder discusses the signs, symptoms, and treatment of chronic illnesses and conditions often linked to anxiety, such as attention deficit hyperactivity disorder (ADHD), bipolar disorder, borderline personality disorder (BPD), depression, eating disorders, illness anxiety disorder, obsessive-compulsive disorder (OCD), post-traumatic stress disorder (PTSD), somatic symptom disorder, substance-use disorder, and suicidal ideation.

Part 5: Lifestyle Modifications for Mental Health and Well-Being describes how one can manage and cope with the symptoms of anxiety. It discusses how diet and physical activity help in managing anxiety disorders and provides tips to cope with stress. There is also a special mention on how to manage anxiety and stress related to COVID-19.

Part 6: Looking Ahead highlights ways individuals with anxiety disorders can lead productive lives. It explains how family and peer support can help in recovery. It provides details about financial assistance and help available for people with mental-health problems. It also talks about accommodating employees with anxiety disorder and explains how to address stress-related concerns in the workplace.

Part 7: Research on Anxiety Disorders talks about the role of research in improving the understanding and treatment of anxiety disorders. It provides information about several anxiety-related clinical trials and research activities.

Part 8: Additional Help and Information provides a glossary of terms related to anxiety disorders and directories of mental-health resources and organizations for people with anxiety disorders and other mental concerns.

BIBLIOGRAPHIC NOTE

This volume contains documents and excerpts from publications issued by the following U.S. government agencies: Centers for Disease Control and Prevention (CDC); *Eunice Kennedy Shriver* National Institute of Child Health and Human Development (NICHD); Federal Occupational Health (FOH); National Cancer Institute (NCI); National Center for Complementary and Integrative Health (NCCIH); National Center for Posttraumatic Stress Disorder (NCPTSD); National Institute of Mental Health (NIMH); National Institute on Alcohol Abuse and Alcoholism (NIAAA); National Institute on Drug Abuse (NIDA); National Institute on Drug Abuse (NIDA) for Teens; National Institutes of Health (NIH); *NIH News in Health*; Office of the Assistant Secretary for Preparedness and Response (ASPR); Office on Women's Health (OWH); Substance Abuse and Mental Health Services Administration (SAMHSA); U.S. Department of Health and Human Services (HHS); U.S. Department of Labor (DOL); U.S. Department of Veterans Affairs (VA); U.S. Equal Employment Opportunity Commission (EEOC); and Youth.gov.

It may also contain original material produced by Omnigraphics and reviewed by medical consultants.

ABOUT THE *HEALTH REFERENCE SERIES*

The *Health Reference Series* is designed to provide basic medical information for patients, families, caregivers, and the general public. Each volume provides comprehensive coverage on a particular topic. This is especially important for people who may be dealing with a newly diagnosed disease or a chronic disorder in themselves or in a family member. People looking for preventive guidance, information about disease warning signs, medical statistics, and risk factors for health problems will also find answers to their questions in the *Health Reference Series*. The *Series*, however, is not intended to serve as a tool for diagnosing illness, in prescribing treatments, or as a substitute for the physician–patient relationship. All people concerned about medical symptoms or the possibility of disease are encouraged to seek professional care from an appropriate healthcare provider.

A NOTE ABOUT SPELLING AND STYLE

Health Reference Series editors use *Stedman's Medical Dictionary* as an authority for questions related to the spelling of medical terms and *The Chicago Manual of Style* for questions related to grammatical structures, punctuation, and other editorial concerns. Consistent adherence is not always possible, however, because the individual volumes within the *Series* include many documents from a wide variety of different producers, and the editor's primary goal is to present material from each source as accurately as is possible. This sometimes means that information in different chapters or sections may follow other guidelines and alternate spelling authorities. For example, occasionally a copyright holder may require that eponymous terms be shown in possessive forms (Crohn's disease vs. Crohn disease) or that British spelling norms be retained (leukaemia vs. leukemia).

MEDICAL REVIEW

Omnigraphics contracts with a team of qualified, senior medical professionals who serve as medical consultants for the *Health Reference Series*. As necessary, medical consultants review reprinted and originally written material for currency and accuracy. Citations including the phrase "Reviewed (month, year)" indicate material reviewed by this team. Medical consultation services are provided to the *Health Reference Series* editors by:

Dr. Vijayalakshmi, MBBS, DGO, MD
Dr. Senthil Selvan, MBBS, DCH, MD
Dr. K. Sivanandham, MBBS, DCH, MS (Research), PhD

HEALTH REFERENCE SERIES UPDATE POLICY

The inaugural book in the *Health Reference Series* was the first edition of *Cancer Sourcebook* published in 1989. Since then, the *Series* has been enthusiastically received by librarians and in the medical community. In order to maintain the standard of providing high-quality health information for the layperson the editorial staff at Omnigraphics felt it was necessary to implement a policy of updating volumes when warranted.

Medical researchers have been making tremendous strides, and it is the purpose of the *Health Reference Series* to stay current with the most recent advances. Each decision to update a volume is made on an individual basis. Some of the considerations include how much new information is available and the feedback we receive from people who use the books. If there is a topic you would like to see added to the update list, or an area of medical concern you feel has not been adequately addressed, please write to:

Managing Editor
Health Reference Series
Omnigraphics
615 Griswold St., Ste. 520
Detroit, MI 48226

Part 1 | Introduction to Mental-Health and Anxiety Disorders

Chapter 1 | Introduction to Mental-Health Disorders

Chapter Contents

Section 1.1 | What Is Mental Health?

This section includes text excerpted from "Learn about Mental Health," Centers for Disease Control and Prevention (CDC), January 26, 2018.

WHAT IS MENTAL ILLNESS?

Mental illnesses are conditions that affect a person's thinking, feeling, mood, or behavior such as depression, anxiety, bipolar disorder, or schizophrenia. Such conditions may be occasional or long-lasting (chronic) and affect someone's ability to relate to others and function each day.

WHAT IS MENTAL HEALTH?

Mental health includes a person's emotional, psychological, and social well-being. It affects how we think, feel, and act. It also helps determine how we handle stress, relate to others, and make healthy choices. Mental health is important at every stage of life, from childhood and adolescence through adulthood.

Although the terms are often used interchangeably, poor mental health and mental illness are not the same things. A person can experience poor mental health and not be diagnosed with a mental illness. Likewise, a person diagnosed with a mental illness can experience periods of physical, mental, and social well-being.

WHY IS MENTAL HEALTH IMPORTANT FOR OVERALL HEALTH?

Mental and physical health are equally important components of overall health. Mental illness, especially depression, increases the risk for many types of physical health problems, particularly long-lasting conditions such as stroke, type 2 diabetes, and heart disease. Similarly, the presence of chronic conditions can increase the risk of mental illness.

CAN YOUR MENTAL HEALTH CHANGE OVER TIME?

Yes, it is important to remember that a person's mental health can change over time, depending on many factors. When the demands placed on a person exceed their resources and coping abilities, their mental health could be impacted. For example, if someone is working long hours, caring for an ill relative, or experiencing economic hardship they may experience poor mental health.

HOW COMMON ARE MENTAL ILLNESSES?

Mental illnesses are among the most common health conditions in the United States.

- More than 50 percent are diagnosed with a mental illness or disorder at some point in their lifetime.
- 1 in 5 Americans will experience a mental illness in a given year.
- 1 in 5 children, either currently or at some point during their life, have had a seriously debilitating mental illness.
- 1 in 25 Americans lives with a serious mental illness such as schizophrenia, bipolar disorder, or major depression.

WHAT CAUSES MENTAL ILLNESS

There is no single cause for mental illness. A number of factors can contribute to risk for mental illness, such as:

- Early adverse life experiences, such as trauma or a history of abuse (e.g., child abuse, sexual assault, witnessing violence, etc.)
- Experiences related to other ongoing (chronic) medical conditions, such as cancer or diabetes
- Biological factors, such as genes or chemical imbalances in the brain
- Use of alcohol or recreational drugs
- Having few friends
- Having a feeling of loneliness or isolation

Section 1.2 | **Mental-Health Myths and Facts**

This section includes text excerpted from "Mental Health Myths and Facts," MentalHealth.gov, U.S. Department of Health and Human Services (HHS), August 29, 2017.

MENTAL-HEALTH PROBLEMS AFFECT EVERYONE

Myth: Mental-health problems do not affect me.

Fact: Mental-health problems are actually very common. In 2014, about:

- One in 5 American adults experienced a mental-health issue
- One in 10 young people experienced a period of major depression
- One in 25 Americans lived with a serious mental illness such as schizophrenia, bipolar disorder, or major depression

Suicide is the tenth leading cause of death in the United States. It accounts for the loss of more than 41,000 American lives each year, more than double the number of lives lost to homicide.

Myth: Children do not experience mental-health problems.

Fact: Even young children may show early warning signs of mental-health concerns. These mental-health problems are often clinically diagnosable and can be a product of the interaction of biological, psychological, and social factors.

Half of all mental-health disorders show first signs before a person turns 14 years of age, and three-quarters of mental-health disorders begin before 24 years of age.

Unfortunately, less than 20 percent of children and adolescents with diagnosable mental-health problems receive the treatment they need. Early mental-health support can help a child before problems interfere with other developmental needs.

Myth: People with mental-health problems are violent and unpredictable.

Fact: The vast majority of people with mental-health problems are no more likely to be violent than anyone else. Most people with mental illness are not violent and only 3 to 5 percent of violent acts can be attributed to individuals living with a serious mental illness. In fact, people with severe mental illnesses are over 10 times more likely to be victims of violent crime than the general population. You probably know someone with a mental-health problem and do not even realize it, because many people with mental-health problems are highly active and productive members of our communities.

Myth: People with mental-health needs, even those who are managing their mental illness, cannot tolerate the stress of holding down a job.

Fact: People with mental-health problems are just as productive as other employees. Employers who hire people with mental-health problems report good attendance and punctuality as well as motivation, good work, and job tenure on par with or greater than other employees.

When employees with mental-health problems receive effective treatment, it can result in:

- Lower total medical costs
- Increased productivity
- Lower absenteeism
- Decreased disability costs

Myth: Personality weakness or character flaws cause mental-health problems. People with mental-health problems can snap out of it if they try hard enough.

Fact: Mental-health problems have nothing to do with being lazy or weak and many people need help to get better. Many factors contribute to mental-health problems, including:

- Biological factors such as genes, physical illness, injury, or brain chemistry
- Life experiences, such as trauma or a history of abuse
- Family history of mental-health problems

People with mental-health problems can get better and many recover completely.

HELPING INDIVIDUALS WITH MENTAL-HEALTH PROBLEMS

Myth: There is no hope for people with mental-health problems. Once a friend or family member develops mental-health problems, she or he will never recover.

Fact: Studies show that people with mental-health problems get better and many recover completely. "Recovery" refers to the process in which people are able to live, work, learn, and participate fully in their communities. There are more treatments, services, and community support systems than ever before, and they work.

Myth: Therapy and self-help are a waste of time. Why bother when you can just take a pill?

Fact: Treatment for mental-health problems varies depending on the individual and could include medication, therapy, or both. Many individuals work with a support system during the healing and recovery process.

Myth: I cannot do anything for a person with a mental-health problem.

Fact: Friends and loved ones can make a big difference. Only 44 percent of adults with diagnosable mental-health problems and less than 20 percent of children and adolescents receive needed treatment. Friends and family can be important influences to help someone get the treatment and services they need by:

- Reaching out and letting them know you are available to help
- Helping them access mental-health services
- Learning and sharing the facts about mental health, especially if you hear something that is not true
- Treating them with respect, just as you would anyone else
- Refusing to define them by their diagnosis or using labels, such as "crazy"

Myth: Prevention does not work. It is impossible to prevent mental illnesses.

Fact: Prevention of mental, emotional, and behavioral disorders focuses on addressing known risk factors, such as exposure to trauma that can affect the chances that children, youth, and young adults will develop mental-health problems. Promoting the social and emotional well-being of children and youth leads to:

- Higher overall productivity
- Better educational outcomes

- Lower crime rates
- Stronger economies
- Lower healthcare costs
- Improved quality of life (QOL)
- Increased lifespan
- Improved family life

Chapter 2 | **Understanding Anxiety Disorders**

Many of us worry from time to time. We fret over finances, feel anxious about job interviews, or get nervous about social gatherings. These feelings can be normal or even helpful. They may give us a boost of energy or help us focus. But, for people with anxiety disorders, they can be overwhelming.

WHEN PANIC, FEAR, AND WORRIES OVERWHELM

Anxiety disorders affect nearly 1 in 5 American adults each year. People with these disorders have feelings of fear and uncertainty that interfere with everyday activities and last for 6 months or more. Anxiety disorders can also raise your risk for other medical problems such as heart disease, diabetes, substance abuse, and depression.

The good news is that most anxiety disorders get better with therapy. The course of treatment depends on the type of anxiety disorder. Medications, psychotherapy ("talk therapy"), or a combination of both can usually relieve troubling symptoms.

"Anxiety disorders are one of the most treatable mental-health problems we see," says Dr. Daniel Pine, a National Institutes of Health (NIH) neuroscientist and psychiatrist. "Still, for reasons we do not fully understand, most people who have these problems do not get the treatments that could really help them."

One of the most common types of anxiety disorder is social anxiety disorder, also known as "social phobia." It affects both women

This chapter includes text excerpted from "Understanding Anxiety Disorders: When Panic, Fear, and Worries Overwhelm," *NIH News in Health*, National Institutes of Health (NIH), March 2016. Reviewed August 2020.

and men equally—a total of about 15 million U.S. adults. Without treatment, social phobia can last for years or even a lifetime. People with social phobia may worry for days or weeks before a social event. They are often embarrassed, self-conscious, and afraid of being judged. They find it hard to talk to others. They may blush, sweat, tremble, or feel sick to their stomach when around other people.

Other common types of anxiety disorders include generalized anxiety disorder (GAD), which affects nearly 7 million American adults, and panic disorder, which affects about 6 million. Both are twice as common in women as in men.

People with GAD worry endlessly over everyday issues—such as health, money, or family problems—even if they realize there is little cause for concern. They startle easily, cannot relax, and cannot concentrate. They find it hard to fall asleep or stay asleep. They may get headaches, muscle aches, or unexplained pains. Symptoms often get worse during times of stress.

People with panic disorder have sudden, repeated bouts of fear—called "panic attacks"—that last several minutes or more. During a panic attack, they may feel that they cannot breathe or that they are having a heart attack. They may fear the loss of control or feel a sense of unreality. Not everyone who has panic attacks will develop panic disorder. But, if the attacks recur without warning, creating fear of having another attack at any time, then it is likely a panic disorder.

Anxiety disorders tend to run in families. But, researchers are not certain why some family members develop these conditions while others do not. No specific genes have been found to actually cause an anxiety disorder. "Many different factors—including genes, stress, and the environment—have small effects that add up in complex ways to affect a person's risk for these disorders," Pine says.

"Many kids with anxiety disorders will outgrow their conditions. But, most anxiety problems we see in adults started during their childhood," Pine adds.

"Anxiety disorders are among the most common psychiatric disorders in children, with an estimated 1 in 3 suffering anxiety at some point during childhood or adolescence," says Dr. Susan Whitfield-Gabrieli, a brain imaging expert at the Massachusetts Institute of Technology. "About half of diagnosable mental-health disorders start by 14 years of age, so there is a lot of interest in uncovering the factors that might influence the brain by those early teen years."

Whitfield-Gabrieli is launching an NIH-funded study to create detailed magnetic resonance imaging (MRI) images of the brains of more than 200 teens, 14 to 15 years of age, with and without anxiety or depression. The scientists will then assess what brain structures and activities might be linked to these conditions. The study is part of the NIH's Human Connectome Project, in which research teams across the country are studying the complex brain connections that affect health and disease.

Whitfield-Gabrieli and colleagues have shown that analysis of brain connections might help predict which adults with social phobia will likely respond to cognitive-behavioral therapy (CBT). CBT is a type of talk therapy known to be effective for people with anxiety disorders. It helps them change their thinking patterns and how they react to anxiety-provoking situations. But, it does not work for everyone.

Of 38 adults with social phobia, those who responded best after three months of CBT had similar patterns of brain connections. This brain analysis led to major improvement, compared to a clinician's assessment alone, in predicting treatment response. Larger studies will be needed to confirm the benefits of the approach.

"Ultimately, we hope that brain imaging will help us predict clinical outcomes and actually tailor the treatment to each individual—to know whether they will respond best to psychotherapy or to certain medications," Whitfield-Gabrieli says.

Other researches are focusing on our emotions and our ability to adjust them. "We want to understand not only how emotions can help us but also how they can create difficulties if they are of the wrong intensity or the wrong type for a particular situation," says Dr. James Gross, a clinical psychologist at Stanford University.

We all use different strategies to adjust our emotions, often without thinking about it. If something makes you angry, you may try to tamp down your emotion to avoid making a scene. If something annoys you, you might try to ignore it, modify it, or entirely avoid it.

But, these strategies can turn harmful over time. For instance, people with social phobia might decide to avoid attending a professional conference so they can keep their anxiety in check. That makes them lose opportunities at work and miss chances to meet people and make friends.

Gross and others are examining the differences between how people with and without anxiety disorders regulate their emotions. "We are finding that CBT is helpful in part because it teaches people to more effectively use emotion regulation strategies," Gross says. "They then become more competent in their ability to use these strategies in their everyday lives."

"It is important to be aware that many different kinds of treatments are available, and people with anxiety disorders tend to have very good responses to those treatments," Pine adds. The best way to start is often by talking with your physician. If you are a parent, talk with your child's pediatrician. "These health professionals are generally prepared to help identify such problems and help patients get the appropriate care they need," Pine says.

Chapter 3 | Brain Circuits Involved in Fear and Anxiety Disorders

Mental disorders are common. You may have a friend, colleague, or relative with a mental disorder, or perhaps you have experienced one yourself at some point. Such disorders include depression, anxiety disorders, bipolar disorder, attention deficit hyperactivity disorder (ADHD), and many others.

Some people who develop a mental illness may recover completely; others may have repeated episodes of illness with relatively stable periods in between. Still, others live with symptoms of mental illness every day. They can be moderate, or serious and cause severe disability.

Through research, it is known that mental disorders are brain disorders. Evidence shows that they can be related to changes in the anatomy, physiology, and chemistry of the nervous system. When the brain cannot effectively coordinate the billions of cells in the body, the results can affect many aspects of life. Scientists are continually learning more about how the brain grows and works in healthy people, and how normal brain development and function can go awry, leading to mental illnesses.

This chapter includes text excerpted from "Brain Basics," National Institute of Mental Health (NIMH), July 5, 2016. Reviewed August 2020.

INSIDE THE BRAIN: NEURONS AND NEURAL CIRCUITS

Neurons are the basic working unit of the brain and nervous system. These cells are highly specialized for the function of conducting messages. A neuron has three basic parts:

- **Cell body,** which includes the nucleus, cytoplasm, and cell organelles. The nucleus contains deoxyribonucleic acid (DNA) and information that the cell needs for growth, metabolism, and repair. The cytoplasm is the substance that fills a cell, including all the chemicals and parts needed for the cell to work properly including small structures called "cell organelles."
- **Dendrites** branch off from the cell body and act as a neuron's point of contact for receiving chemical and electrical signals called "impulses" from neighboring neurons.
- **Axon,** which sends impulses and extends from cell bodies to meet and deliver impulses to another nerve cell. Axons can range in length from a fraction of an inch to several feet.

Each neuron is enclosed by a cell membrane, which separates the inside contents of the cell from its surrounding environment and controls what enters and leaves the cell, and responds to signals from the environment; this all helps the cell maintain its balance with the environment.

Synapses are tiny gaps between neurons, where messages move from one neuron to another as chemical or electrical signals.

The brain begins as a small group of cells in the outer layer of a developing embryo. As the cells grow and differentiate, neurons travel from a central "birthplace" to their final destination. Chemical signals from other cells guide neurons in forming various brain structures. Neighboring neurons make connections with each other and with distant nerve cells (via axons) to form brain circuits. These circuits control specific body functions such as sleep and speech. The brain continues maturing well into a person's early 20s. Knowing how the brain is wired and how the normal brain's structure develops and matures helps scientists understand what goes wrong in mental illnesses.

Scientists have already begun to chart how the brain develops over time in healthy people and are working to compare that with brain development in people with mental disorders. Genes and environmental cues both help to direct this growth.

NEUROTRANSMITTERS

Everything we do relies on neurons communicating with one another. Electrical impulses and chemical signals carrying messages across different parts of the brain and between the brain and the rest of the nervous system.

When a neuron is activated a small difference in electrical charge occurs. This unbalanced charge is called an "action potential" and is caused by the concentration of ions (atoms or molecules with unbalanced charges) across the cell membrane. The action potential travels very quickly along the axon, such as when a line of dominoes falls.

When the action potential reaches the end of an axon, most neurons release a chemical message (a neurotransmitter) that crosses the synapse and binds to receptors on the receiving neuron's dendrites and starts the process over again. At the end of the line, a neurotransmitter may stimulate a different kind of cell (such as a gland cell) or may trigger a new chain of messages.

Neurotransmitters send chemical messages between neurons. Mental illnesses, such as depression, can occur when this process does not work correctly. Communication between neurons can also be electrical, such as in areas of the brain that control movement. When electrical signals are abnormal, they can cause tremors or symptoms found in Parkinson disease.

- **Serotonin**—helps control many functions, such as mood, appetite, and sleep. Research shows that people with depression often have lower than normal levels of serotonin. The types of medications most commonly prescribed to treat depression act by blocking the recycling, or reuptake of serotonin by the sending neuron. As a result, more serotonin stays in the synapse for the receiving neuron to bind onto, leading to more normal mood functioning.

- **Dopamine**—mainly involved in controlling movement and aiding the flow of information to the front of the brain, which is linked to thought and emotion. It is also linked to reward systems in the brain. Problems in producing dopamine can result in Parkinson disease, a disorder that affects a person's ability to move as they want to, resulting in stiffness, tremors or shaking, and other symptoms. Some studies suggest that having too little dopamine or problems using dopamine in the thinking and feeling regions of the brain may play a role in disorders such as schizophrenia or attention deficit hyperactivity disorder (ADHD).
- **Glutamate**—the most common neurotransmitter, glutamate has many roles throughout the brain and nervous system. Glutamate is an excitatory transmitter, when it is released it increases the chance that the neuron will fire. This enhances the electrical flow among brain cells required for normal function and plays an important role during early brain development. It may also assist in learning and memory. Problems in making or using glutamate have been linked to many mental disorders.

BRAIN REGIONS

Just as many neurons working together form a circuit, many circuits work together to form specialized brain systems. We have many specialized brain systems that work across specific brain regions to help us talk, help us make sense of what we see, and help us to solve a problem. Some of the regions most commonly studied in mental-health research are listed below.

- **Amygdala**—The brain's "fear hub," which activates our natural "fight-or-flight" response to confront or escape from a dangerous situation. The amygdala also appears to be involved in learning to fear an event, such as touching a hot stove and learning not to fear, such as overcoming a fear of spiders. Studying how the amygdala helps create memories of fear and safety may help improve treatments for anxiety disorders like phobias or posttraumatic stress disorder (PTSD).

- **Prefrontal cortex (PFC)**—Seat of the brain's executive functions, such as judgment, decision making, and problem-solving. Different parts of the PFC are involved in using short-term or "working" memory and in retrieving long-term memories. This area of the brain also helps to control the amygdala during stressful events. Some research shows that people who have PTSD or ADHD have reduced activity in their PFCs.

- **Anterior cingulate cortex (ACC)**—the ACC has many different roles, from controlling blood pressure and heart rate to responding when we sense a mistake, helping us feel motivated and stay focused on a task, and managing proper emotional reactions. Reduced ACC activity or damage to this brain area has been linked to disorders such as ADHD, schizophrenia, and depression.

- **Hippocampus**—Helps create and file new memories. When the hippocampus is damaged, a person cannot create new memories, but can still remember past events and learned skills, and carry on a conversation, all of which rely on different parts of the brain. The hippocampus may be involved in mood disorders through its control of a major mood circuit called the "hypothalamic-pituitary-adrenal" (HPA) axis.

Chapter 4 | Potential Risk Factors for Anxiety Disorder

Chapter Contents

"Behavioral Inhibition: A Predictor of Anxiety Disorders," © 2020 Omnigraphics. Reviewed August 2020.

BEHAVIORAL INHIBITION

Behavioral inhibition (BI) is a condition that has been associated with the development of social anxiety disorder (SAD). It deals with the tendency to experience distress and withdrawal from unfamiliar situations, persons, or environment. The potential development of anxiety can be determined by examining children with BI. In unfamiliar environment, children with BI tend to be nervous, anxious, uncomfortable, tend to avoid playing, withdraw themselves, and appear to be very aware of their surroundings.

Although research on BI and its efficacy for predicting anxiety later in life is still in its infancy, studies indicate that this could be a significant predictor that would require earlier care. Social anxiety may be a disturbing mental disorder that has severe negative effects. Early detection and intervention are important for improving the quality of life (QOL) and avoiding certain disorders, such as depression.

ANXIETY DISORDER

Although the exact cause of specific anxiety disorders, such as SAD has not been identified by researchers, many believe it is related to genetic and environmental reasons. For years, many people suffer extreme social anxiety without receiving appropriate care, either because they are not seeking support or because they are being treated incorrectly. Anxiety begins for many during their adolescence and young adulthood. The level of anxiety in a person can be reduced by diagnosing it at an early age and giving them the ability to take appropriate treatment options. BI is an important aspect of childhood as it can be an early indicator of anxiety disorders and is valuable for a suitable diagnosis to be made. Untreated anxiety can lead to extreme depression and even suicidal behavior.

RELATIONSHIP BETWEEN BEHAVIORAL INHIBITION AND ANXIETY DISORDER

Researchers have indicated a connection between childhood personality and the development of social anxiety in life. BI is a form of personality that shows a tendency toward nervousness and anxiety. When children grow older, a lot of them tend to adapt more rationally to new circumstances and new people, while a few will continue to exhibit anxious behaviors throughout their lives.

HOW TO DECREASE BEHAVIORAL INHIBITION TO MINIMIZE ANXIETY DISORDER

The BI temperamental construct can be an early identifiable risk factor for anxiety disorders and is therefore useful for targeting at-risk children. In the study of BI and social anxiety, therapists can intervene early to prevent an increase in anxiety level. The effective way to encourage a child to be confident is to encourage them to be independent and allow them the ability to solve issues by themselves. This can build a foundation on which the child in social situations does not need to rely on others, diminishing the chances of developing social anxiety later on.

Over-protective care, such as providing help where it is not needed, may increase behavioral resistance and may raise anxiety in new circumstances. It may encourage the implementation of future prevention interventions aimed at precluding an anxiety disorder from emerging.

References

1. Cuncic, Arlin. "Link Between Behavioral Inhibition and Social Anxiety," Very Well Mind, March 26, 2020.
2. "Behavioral Inhibition as a Childhood Predictor of Social Anxiety," Andrew Kukes Foundation for Social Anxiety, September 7, 2012.
3. Svihra, Martin; Katzman, A Martin. "Behavioral inhibition: A Predictor of Anxiety," National Center for Biotechnology Information, October 15, 2004.

Section 4.2 | **Gender**

This section contains text excerpted from the following sources: Text in this section begins with excerpts from "Women's Mental Health and Gender Differences Research," National Institutes of Health (NIH), March 6, 2000. Reviewed August 2020; Text under the heading "Role of Anxiety Molecules" is excerpted from "Anxiety Molecules Affect Male and Female Mice Differently," National Institutes of Health (NIH), October 25, 2016. Reviewed August 2020; Text under the heading "What Is the Latest Research on Anxiety Disorders and Women?" is excerpted from "Anxiety disorders," Office on Women's Health (OWH), U.S. Department of Health and Human Services (HHS), January 30, 2019.

Of all demographic variables in epidemiological research, gender is the single strongest correlate of risk for different types of mental disorders. Despite the robustness of this correlation, "gender" itself is a proxy term for a complex of biological, behavioral, and psychosocial variables and processes, which remain as yet incompletely understood. Depressive disorders and most anxiety disorders are, on average, two to three times more common in females than males. Eating disorders are eight to ten times more common in females. Males are more likely to be affected by developmental disorders such as autism and attention deficit disorder and by substance and alcohol abuse and conduct disorders. For all disorders, including those more common in males than females and those in which gender prevalence is equal (e.g., schizophrenia, bipolar disorder), gender-related differences may occur in etiological risk factors or in clinical aspects. Gender differences in features such as neuropsychological profiles, the risk for onset or recurrence, symptom severity, or disability have important practical significance for treatment and services needs.

In general, women are the primary consumers of treatments and services for mental disorders, but there is little consideration of epidemiological and clinical findings of gender differences applied to public mental-health policy and services delivery systems.

The majority of serious mental disorders have an onset in early adulthood or adolescence and a recurrent or chronic course. Thus the social impact of mental disorders falls disproportionately on women during the childbearing and childrearing years suggesting the need for more intervention research for women during pregnancy and lactation.

HOW GENDER AFFECTS THE RISK OF DEVELOPING MENTAL DISORDERS

Despite clear gender differences in the prevalence of different mental disorders, there is relatively little linkage between epidemiological, etiological, and intervention research.

There is as yet an imprecise lexicon to describe differences in health status, etiology, progress, and treatment of disease between men and women.

This difficulty reflects persistent conceptual lack of clarity related to the roles of biological, social, and cultural factors in differences. In what follows, the term "gender" is used to refer to multiple processes and factors. However, investigators are encouraged to discuss their conceptual models of gender differences in their applications.

Brain and Behavior Research

There is increased recognition that biologically mediated gender differences influence behavioral outcomes and may modify vulnerability to different mental disorders, the severity of course, or response to different treatments.

Included here are basic studies in animals and humans as well as human clinical studies in subjects with mental disorders.

Bio-Behavioral Dysregulation and Adaptation to Stress

Evidence is accruing that response to stress may be mediated both by sex steroids as well as by experiential differences between men and women. Animal and human studies indicate that gender differences in hormonal factors may modulate physiological and behavioral responses to stress. Epidemiological studies show that women are more likely to have experienced certain kinds of stress (e.g., childhood and adult sexual abuse), which are risk factors for mental disorders. Research also indicates that women are twice as likely as men to develop stress-related disorders and depression following exposure to traumatic events. To understand this complex area, multiple approaches are required, ranging from basic developmental and plasticity research to human clinical studies.

Epidemiological and Clinical Studies of Disorders

During the past two decades, advances in diagnosis and survey methodologies have enabled researchers to establish general estimates of the impact and service needs of adult women with mental disorders. The need for such research is particularly pressing since, in many disorders, gender differences emerge first in adolescence when early intervention strategies may be most effective in preventing full-blown mental disorders. Later in the lifespan, there is relatively little information on gender-related factors in important clinical aspects of disorders such as the risk for recurrence, chronicity, comorbidity, and disability.

Reproductive Transitions

Menarche coincides with the onset of gender disparities in the incidence of depression and eating disorders. Menstruation is associated with severe mood variations in a small percentage of women. Since variance in hormonal levels per se has been found to have little correlation with mood or mood change in human research, there is a need for studies of the interaction of multiple biological, clinical, and environmental factors. Pregnancy and recent childbearing may be associated with higher rates of depressive disorders. This association, as well as the fact that psychotropic drugs are commonly prescribed for women of childbearing age, raises special gender-related clinical and treatment considerations. Bioethical issues in the conduct of clinical research take on added importance since psychotropic agents have the potential to affect the fetus or nursing child.

Other Interventions and Services Research

In addition to interventions targeted specifically for women during reproductive transitions, federally funded phase III clinical trials and phase III submissions to the U.S. Food and Drug Administration (FDA) for approval of new treatments for use in both males and females are required to include sufficient numbers of females to permit analysis of outcome data for gender differences. This general focus also underscores the need to examine interventions for their impact separately in males and females, to identify multiple factors in relation to the outcome and to address issues affecting recruitment and retention of female subjects in trials.

ROLE OF ANXIETY MOLECULES

A team of researchers led by Dr. Nathaniel Heintz at Rockefeller University previously discovered a group of oxytocin-responsive brain cells—called "oxytocin receptor interneurons"—that regulate social behavior in female mice. To investigate possible sex-related differences of these neurons, the researchers genetically inserted a light-activated sensor into the brain cells of both male and female mice. This allowed the scientists to control the activity of the brain cells with light and observe the animals' behavior at the same time.

The scientists activated oxytocin receptor interneurons and then compared how anxious or social the mice were during different tasks. The team measured the animals' behaviors while they explored an open field or an elevated maze or while in a chamber with an unfamiliar mouse of the opposite sex. After the brain cells were activated, male mice became less anxious but the females did not. The female animals did, however, become more social.

The light-activated brain cells project into two areas of the medial prefrontal cortex, a brain region, responsible for complex behaviors. In male mice, cells in one of the areas responded more robustly to the light activation. Cells in this region were also more sensitive in male animals to a stress hormone called "corticotropin-releasing hormone" (CRH). The researchers determined that oxytocin receptor interneurons released a molecule called "corticotropin-releasing hormone binding protein" (CRHBP) that blocked the activity of CRH. CRHBP thus reduced the stress hormone's effect on cells in the male brain. The team found that female mice had higher levels of CRH in their brains. This likely accounts for their lack of sensitivity to CRHBP's stress-reducing effects.

Stress, social situations, and sex-related differences can affect how much oxytocin and CRH are present in different brain areas. It was suggested that the balance between oxytocin and CRH levels may be what determines the differences in behavior.

"Emotional and social behaviors are complicated, so finding any clues to why some people are more vulnerable to anxiety than others, or why some are social while others are not, matters" Heintz says. "These are fundamental questions of human behavior that we do not yet understand fully."

WHAT IS THE LATEST RESEARCH ON ANXIETY DISORDERS AND WOMEN?

Researchers are studying why women are more than twice as likely as men to develop anxiety disorders and depression. Changes in levels of the hormone estrogen throughout a woman's menstrual cycle and reproductive life (during the years a woman can have a baby) probably play a role.

Researchers also studied the male hormone testosterone, which is found in women and men but typically in higher levels in men. They found that treatment with testosterone had similar effects as anti-anxiety and antidepressant medication for the women in the study.

Other research focuses on anxiety disorders and depression during and after pregnancy and among women who are overweight and obese.

Section 4.3 | The Genetic Basis of Anxiety Disorders

This section contains text excerpted from the following sources: Text in this section begins with excerpts from "Looking at My Genes: What Can They Tell Me about My Mental Health?" National Institute of Mental Health (NIMH), 2020; Text beginning with the heading "Million Veteran Program Study Sheds Light on Genetic Basis of Anxiety" is excerpted from "Million Veteran Program Study Sheds Light on Genetic Basis of Anxiety," U.S. Department of Veterans Affairs (VA), January 7, 2020.

Mental disorders are health conditions that affect how a person thinks, feels, and acts. These disorders can impact a person's life in significant ways, including how they cope with life events, earn a living, and relate to others.

"Why did this happen?" That is a common question that patients and their families have following a psychotic episode, a suicide attempt, or the diagnosis of a mental disorder.

Research conducted and funded by the National Institute of Mental Health (NIMH) has found that many mental disorders are caused by a combination of biological, environmental, psychological, and genetic factors. In fact, a growing body of research has found that certain genes and gene variations are associated with mental disorders.

YOUR FAMILY HEALTH HISTORY

Your family health history may be one of your best clues for determining your risk of developing a mental disorder and many other common illnesses. Certain mental disorders tend to run in families, and having a close relative with a mental disorder could mean you are at a higher risk.

If a family member has a mental disorder, it does not necessarily mean you will develop one. Many other factors also play a role. But, knowing your family's mental-health history can help you determine whether you are at a higher risk for certain disorders, help your doctor to recommend actions for reducing your risk, and enable both you and your doctor to look for early warning signs.

To gain a better understanding of your family health history, it may help to talk to your blood relatives, keep a record of your family history, talk with a mental-health professional, or visit a genetic counselor.

CAN GENETIC TESTING HELP PREDICT YOUR RISK OF DEVELOPING A MENTAL DISORDER?

The short answer to this question is no. Currently, genetic tests cannot accurately predict your risk of developing a mental disorder. Although research is underway, scientists do not yet know all the gene variations that contribute to mental disorders, and those that are known, so far, raise the risk by very small amounts.

One day, genetic research may make it possible to provide a more complete picture of a person's risk of getting a particular mental disorder or to diagnose it, based on her or his genes. Although recent studies have begun to identify the genetic markers associated with certain mental disorders and eventually may lead to better screening and more personalized treatment, it is still too early to use genetic tests or genome scans to diagnose or treat mental disorders accurately.

MILLION VETERAN PROGRAM STUDY SHEDS LIGHT ON GENETIC BASIS OF ANXIETY

In the largest genetic study on anxiety to date, VA researchers found new evidence on the underlying biological causes of the disorder. The study used VA Million Veteran Program (MVP) data to identify regions on the human genome related to anxiety risk. This could lead to new understanding and treatment of the condition, which affects one in 10 Americans.

According to Dr. Dan Levey of the VA Connecticut Healthcare Center and Yale University, one of the lead authors on the study, the findings are "an important step forward" in the understanding of anxiety disorders and how genes contribute to mental conditions.

Working toward "Precision Medicine" for Anxiety Disorders

"Anxiety" refers to the anticipation of perceived future threats. In anxiety disorders, these concerns are out of proportion to the actual anticipated event, leading to distress and disability. Anxiety disorders often occur alongside other mental-health disorders such as depression.

Only a third of those with anxiety disorders receive treatment. Some forms of psychotherapy, such as cognitive-behavioral therapy (CBT), have proved effective, as have medications such as selective serotonin reuptake inhibitors (SSRIs). In other fields of medicine, genetic studies have led to precision medicine approaches—tailoring drug treatment to patients' individual genetic and biochemical profiles—for a number of diseases. The researchers hope more genetic insight will lead to similar approaches for anxiety.

The researchers compared the genomes of nearly 200,000 MVP participants. They identified five locations on the human genome related to anxiety in Americans of European descent, and one in African Americans. Gene variants at these genome locations could increase anxiety risk, say the scientists.

The findings for the African-American participants are especially important, says Levey. "Minorities are underrepresented in genetic studies," he wrote in an e-mail, "and the diversity of the Million Veteran Program was essential for this part of the project. The genetic variant we identified occurs only in individuals of African ancestry, and would have been completely missed in less diverse cohorts."

The study produced the first genome-wide significant findings on anxiety in African ancestry, notes Levey. About 18 percent of MVP participants are African American.

The anxiety-related genome locations also show overlap with other psychiatric conditions. One of the identified locations has previously been linked with risk for bipolar disorder and schizophrenia. The study also shows a genetic overlap between anxiety symptoms and depression, PTSD (which is related to anxiety), and neuroticism—a personality trait that has been shown to increase the risk for anxiety and related disorders. The results support the idea that overlap with these other traits is at least partially due to a significant genetic commonality, according to the researchers.

Section 4.4 | Epigenetic Interaction in Psychiatric Disorders

This section contains text excerpted from the following sources: Text in this section begins with excerpts from "Brain Basics," National Institute of Mental Health (NIMH), July 5, 2016. Reviewed August 2020; Text under the heading "Study Finds Epigenetic Changes in Children of Holocaust Survivors" is excerpted from "Study Finds Epigenetic Changes in Children of Holocaust Survivors," U.S. Department of Veterans Affairs (VA), October 26, 2016. Reviewed August 2020.

There are many different types of cells in the body. It is said that cells differentiate as the embryo develops, becoming more specialized for specific functions. Skin cells protect, muscle cells contract, and neurons, the most highly specialized cells of all, conduct messages. Every cell in our bodies contains a complete set of deoxyribonucleic acid (DNA). DNA, the "recipe of life," contains all the information inherited from our parents that helps to define who we are, such as our looks, and certain abilities such as a good singing voice. A gene is a segment of DNA that contains codes to make proteins and other important body chemicals. DNA also includes information to control which genes are expressed and when in all the cells of the body. As we grow, we create new cells, each with a copy of our original set of DNA. Sometimes this copying process is imperfect, leading to a gene mutation that causes the gene to code for a slightly different protein. Some mutations are harmless, some can be helpful, and others give rise to disabilities or diseases.

Genes are not the only determinants of how our bodies function. Throughout our lives, our genes can be affected by the environment. In medicine, the term "environment" includes not only our physical surroundings but also factors that can affect our bodies, such as sleep, diet, or stress. These factors may act alone or together in complex ways, to change the way a gene is expressed or the way messages are conducted in the body.

Epigenetics is the study of how environmental factors can affect how a given gene operates. But, unlike gene mutations, epigenetic changes do not change the code for a gene. Rather, they affect when a gene turns on or off to produce a specific protein. Scientists believe epigenetics plays a major role in mental disorders and the effects of medications. Some, but not all mutations and epigenetic changes can be passed onto future generations. Further understanding of genes and epigenetics may one day lead to genetic testing for people at risk for mental disorders. This could greatly help in early detection, more tailored treatments, and possibly prevention of such illnesses.

STUDY FINDS EPIGENETIC CHANGES IN CHILDREN OF HOLOCAUST SURVIVORS

Dr. Rachel Yehuda, a neuroscientist at the James J. Peters Veterans Affairs Medical Center in the Bronx, New York, has spent decades studying the biological roots of posttraumatic stress disorder (PTSD) in relation to Veterans, Holocaust survivors, and other trauma victims.

She and her colleagues showed for the first time in humans that epigenetic changes caused by exposure to trauma can be passed on to children born after the event—in this case, Holocaust survivors and their adult children. Epigenetic processes alter the expression of a gene without producing changes in the DNA sequence and can be transmitted to the next generation.

Children Show Signs of Depression, Anxiety

Her study yields insight into how severe psychophysiological trauma can have intergenerational effects. "These observations suggest that parental trauma is a relevant contributor to offspring biology," Yehuda says.

The researchers focused on *FKBP5*, a stress gene linked to PTSD, depression, and mood and anxiety disorders. The results suggest that Holocaust exposure had an effect on *FKBP5* methylation—a mechanism that controls the gene's expression—that was observed in parents exposed to the horrors of the concentration camps, as well as their offspring, many of whom showed signs of depression and anxiety.

The research, Yehuda says, did not demonstrate "transmission" of PTSD, only that the parent's experience is somehow related to their offspring's phenotype and biology. Phenotype is an organism's physical appearance and behavior, as determined by genetic and environmental influences.

"The message of the study is that we respond to our environments in multiple ways that can have long-lasting, transformative effects," Yehuda says. "The implications are that what happens to our parents, or perhaps even to our grandparents or previous generations, may help shape who we are on a fundamental molecular level that contributes to our behaviors, beliefs, strengths, and vulnerabilities."

Children of Survivors Struggle with Anxiety More than with Depression, PTSD

Research from a team that involved a the U.S Department of Veterans Affairs (VA) researcher finds that children of Holocaust survivors are experiencing generalized anxiety disorder (GAD)—a condition marked by excessive, uncontrollable, and irrational worry—more than depression and PTSD.

In a study that included interviews with 190 adult children of Holocaust survivors, 18.4 percent reported having GAD in the past year, compared with 13.7 percent for a major depression episode (MDE), and 7.4 percent for PTSD. The study cites 2008 research in noting that the past-year percentage of adults with those conditions in the United States and Israel is much lower: 3.1 (GAD), 6.7 (MDE), and 3.5 (PTSD) in the United States; and 1.8 (GAD), 5.9 (MDE), and 0.5 (PTSD) in Israel.

Researchers for the study say the findings must be taken with "caution" in part because only 190 people were interviewed. However, the results suggest that attention has been disproportionately focused on PTSD for children of Holocaust survivors as opposed to anxiety, the researchers say.

"That GAD was more frequent than PTSD among these children of survivors makes clinical sense," the researchers write. "The parents were directly traumatized by their Holocaust and post-Holocaust experiences. The children were exposed not to the traumas themselves but to their parents' stories and their aftermath, including among others, the message that the world is a dangerous place where the children must be on guard against threats, big and small."

Section 4.5 | Negative Life Events in Early Childhood or Adulthood

This section contains text excerpted from the following sources: Text beginning with the heading "What Is Child Traumatic Stress?" is excerpted from "What Is Child Traumatic Stress?" Substance Abuse and Mental Health Services Administration (SAMHSA), May 12, 2018; Text under the heading "The Three "E's" of Trauma: Event(s), Experience of Event(s), and Effect" is excerpted from "SAMHSA's Concept of Trauma and Guidance for a Trauma-Informed Approach," Substance Abuse and Mental Health Services Administration (SAMHSA), July 15, 2014. Reviewed August 2020.

WHAT IS CHILD TRAUMATIC STRESS?

From a psychological perspective, trauma occurs when a child experiences an intense event that threatens or causes harm to her or his emotional and physical well-being.

Trauma can be the result of exposure to a natural disaster such as a hurricane or flood or to events such as war and terrorism.

Witnessing or being the victim of violence, serious injury, or physical or sexual abuse can be traumatic. Accidents or medical procedures can result in trauma, too. Sadly, about one of every four children will experience a traumatic event before the age of 16.

HOW DOES IT DEVELOP?

When children have a traumatic experience, they react in both physiological and psychological ways. Their heart rate may increase, and they may begin to sweat, to feel agitated and hyperalert, to feel "butterflies" in their stomach, and to become emotionally upset. These reactions are distressing, but in fact, they are normal—they are our bodies' way of protecting us and preparing us to confront danger. However, some children who have experienced a traumatic event will have long-lasting reactions that can interfere with their physical and emotional health.

Children who suffer from child traumatic stress are those children who have been exposed to one or more traumas over the course of their lives and develop reactions that persist and affect their daily lives after the traumatic events have ended. Traumatic reactions can include a variety of responses, including intense and ongoing emotional upset, depressive symptoms, anxiety, behavioral changes, difficulties with attention, academic difficulties, nightmares, physical symptoms such as difficulty sleeping and eating, and aches and pains, among others.

SYMPTOMS OF CHILD TRAUMATIC STRESS

Children who suffer from traumatic stress often have these types of symptoms when reminded in some way of the traumatic event. Although many of us may experience these reactions from time to time, when a child is experiencing child traumatic stress, they interfere with the child's daily life and ability to function and interact with others.

Some of these children may develop ongoing symptoms that are diagnosed as posttraumatic stress disorder (PTSD). When we talk about child traumatic stress, we are talking about the stress of any child who has had a traumatic experience and is having difficulties moving forward with her or his life. When we talk about PTSD, we are talking about a disorder defined by the American Psychiatric Association (APA) as having specific symptoms: the child continues to re-experience the event through nightmares, flashbacks, or other symptoms for more than a month after the original experience; the child has what we call avoidance or numbing symptoms—she or he would not think about the event, has memory lapses, or maybe feels numb in connection with the events—and the child has feelings of arousal, such as increased irritability, difficulty sleeping, or others.

Every child diagnosed with PTSD is experiencing child traumatic stress, but not every child experiencing child traumatic stress has all the symptoms for a PTSD diagnosis. And not every child who experiences a traumatic event will develop symptoms of child traumatic stress. Whether or not your child does, depends on a range of factors. These include her or his history of previous trauma exposure because children who have experienced prior traumas are more likely to develop symptoms after a recent event. They also include an individual child's mental and emotional strengths and weaknesses and what kind of support she or he has at home and elsewhere. Children are unique individuals, and it is unwise to make sweeping assumptions about whether they will or will not experience ongoing troubles following a traumatic event.

For children who do experience traumatic stress, there is a wide variety of potential consequences. In addition to causing the symptoms listed, the experience can have a direct impact on the development of children's brains and bodies. Traumatic stress can interfere with children's ability to concentrate, learn, and perform in school. It can change how children view the world and their futures and can lead to future employment problems. It can also take a tremendous toll on the entire family.

THE THREE "E'S" OF TRAUMA: EVENT(S), EXPERIENCE OF EVENT(S), AND EFFECT

Events and circumstances may include the actual or extreme threat of physical or psychological harm (i.e., natural disasters, violence, etc.) or severe life-threatening neglect for a child that imperils healthy development. These events and circumstances may occur as a single occurrence or repeatedly over time.

The individual's experience of these events or circumstances helps to determine whether it is a traumatic event. A particular event may be experienced as traumatic for one individual and not for another (e.g., a child removed from abusive home experiences this differently than their sibling; one refugee may experience fleeing one's country differently from another refugee; one military veteran may experience deployment to a war zone as traumatic while another veteran is not similarly affected). How the individual labels, assigns meaning to and is disrupted physically and psychologically by an event will contribute to whether or not it is experienced as traumatic. Traumatic events by their very nature set up a power differential where one entity (whether an individual, an event, or a force of nature) has power over another. They elicit a profound question of "why me?" The individual's experience of these events or circumstances is shaped in the context of this powerlessness and questioning.

Feelings of humiliation, guilt, shame, betrayal, or silencing often shaper the experience of the event. When a person experiences physical or sexual abuse, it is often accompanied by a sense of humiliation, which can lead the person to feel as though they are bad or dirty, leading to a sense of self-blame, shame, and guilt. In case of war or natural disasters, those who survived the traumatic event may blame themselves for surviving when others did not. Abuse by a trusted caregiver frequently gives rise to feelings of betrayal, shattering a person's trust and leaving them feeling alone. Often, abuse of children and domestic violence are accompanied by threats that lead to silencing and fear of reaching out for help.

How the event is experienced may be linked to a range of factors including the individual's cultural beliefs (e.g., the subjugation of women and the experience of domestic violence), availability of social support (e.g., whether isolated or embedded in a supportive family or community structure), or to the developmental stage of the individual (i.e., an individual may understand and experience events differently at age five, fifteen, or fifty).

Potential Risk Factors for Anxiety Disorder

The long-lasting adverse effects of the event are a critical component of trauma. These adverse effects may occur immediately or may have a delayed onset. The duration of the effects can be short- or long- term. In some situations, the individual may not recognize the connection between traumatic events and their effects. Examples of adverse effects include an individual's inability to cope with the normal stresses and strains of daily living; to trust and benefit from the relationship; to manage cognitive processes, such as memory, attention, thinking; to regulate behavior; or to control the expression of emotions. In addition to these more visible effects, there may be an altering of one's neurobiological make-up and ongoing health and well-being. Advances in neuroscience and an increased understanding of the interaction of neurobiological and environmental factors have documented the effects of such threatening events. Traumatic effects, which may range from hypervigilance or a constant state of arousal to numbing or avoidance, can eventually wear a person down, physically, mentally, and emotionally. Survivors of trauma have also highlighted the impact of these events on spiritual beliefs and the capacity to make meaning of these experiences.

Chapter 5 | Anxiety Disorder in Specific Populations

Chapter Contents

Section 5.1 | **Anxiety and Depression among Children**

This section includes text excerpted from "Anxiety and Depression in Children," Centers for Disease Control and Prevention (CDC), March 30, 2020.

Many children have fears and worries and may feel sad and hopeless from time to time. Strong fears may appear at different times during development. For example, toddlers are often very distressed about being away from their parents, even if they are safe and cared for. Although fears and worries are typical in children, persistent or extreme forms of fear and sadness could be due to anxiety or depression. Because the symptoms primarily involve thoughts and feelings, they are called "internalizing disorders."

ANXIETY

When a child does not outgrow the fears and worries that are typical in young children, or when there are so many fears and worries that they interfere with school, home, or play activities, the child may be diagnosed with an anxiety disorder. Examples of different types of anxiety disorders include:
- Being very afraid when away from parents (separation anxiety)
- Having extreme fear about a specific thing or situation such as dogs, insects, or going to the doctor (phobias)
- Being very afraid of school and other places where there are people (social anxiety)
- Being very worried about the future and about bad things happening (general anxiety)
- Having repeated episodes of sudden, unexpected, intense fear that come with symptoms such as heart-pounding, having trouble breathing, or feeling dizzy, shaky, or sweaty (panic disorder)

Anxiety may present as fear or worry, but can also make children irritable and angry. Anxiety symptoms can also include trouble sleeping, as well as physical symptoms such as fatigue, headaches, or stomachaches. Some anxious children keep their worries to themselves and, thus, the symptoms can be missed.

DEPRESSION

Some children feel sad or uninterested in things that they used to enjoy or feel helpless or hopeless in situations they are able to change. When children feel persistent sadness and hopelessness, they may be diagnosed with depression.

Examples of behaviors often seen in children with depression include:

- Feeling sad, hopeless, or irritable a lot of the time
- Not wanting to do or enjoy doing fun things
- Showing changes in eating patterns—eating a lot more or a lot less than usual
- Showing changes in sleep patterns—sleeping a lot more or a lot less than normal
- Showing changes in energy—being tired and sluggish or tense and restless a lot of the time
- Having a hard time paying attention
- Feeling worthless, useless, or guilty
- Showing self-injury and self-destructive behavior

Extreme depression can lead a child to think about suicide or plan for suicide. For youth 10 to 24 years of age, suicide is among the leading causes of death.

Some children may not talk about their helpless and hopeless thoughts, and may not appear sad. Depression might also cause a child to make trouble or act unmotivated, causing others not to notice that the child is depressed or to incorrectly label the child as a trouble-maker or lazy.

PREVENTION OF ANXIETY AND DEPRESSION

It is not known exactly why some children develop anxiety or depression. Many factors may play a role, including biology and temperament. But, it is also known that some children are more likely to develop anxiety or depression when they experience trauma or stress, when they are maltreated, when they are bullied or rejected by other children, or when their own parents have anxiety or depression.

Although these factors appear to increase the risk of anxiety or depression, there are ways to decrease the chance that children experience them.

Section 5.2 | **Anxiety among Teens**

This section contains text excerpted from the following sources: Text in this section begins with excerpts from "Mental Health in Adolescents," U.S. Department of Health and Human Services (HHS), May 14, 2020; Text under the heading "How Anxiety Disorders Affect Adolescents" is excerpted from "Common Mental Health Disorders in Adolescence," U.S. Department of Health and Human Services (HHS), May 1, 2019; Text under the heading "U.S. Children and Adolescents with Diagnosed Anxiety and Depression" is excerpted from "Key Findings: U.S. Children with Diagnosed Anxiety and Depression," Centers for Disease Control and Prevention (CDC), March 12, 2019; Text under the heading "Impact of Mental-Health Problems in Adolescence" is excerpted from "Adolescent Mental Health Basics," U.S. Department of Health and Human Services (HHS), May 14, 2020.

Important mental-health habits—including coping, resilience, and good judgment—help adolescents to achieve overall well-being and set the stage for positive mental health in adulthood. Mood swings are common during adolescence. However, some adolescents will experience a serious mental-health disorder, such as depression and/or anxiety disorders, at some point in their life. Friends and family can watch for warning signs of mental disorders and urge young people to get help. Effective treatments exist and may involve a combination of psychotherapy and medication.

HOW ANXIETY DISORDERS AFFECT ADOLESCENTS

- Characterized by feelings of excessive uneasiness, worry, and fear
- Occur in approximately 32 percent of 13- to 18-year-olds
- Examples include:
  - Generalized anxiety disorder (GAD)
  - Posttraumatic stress disorder (PTSD)
  - Social anxiety disorder (SAD)

- Obsessive-compulsive disorder (OCD)
- Phobias

U.S. CHILDREN AND ADOLESCENTS WITH DIAGNOSED ANXIETY AND DEPRESSION

In an article published in the *Journal of Developmental and Behavioral Pediatrics*, the Centers for Disease Control and Prevention (CDC) researchers found that, as of 2011–12, more than 1 in 20, or 2.6 million, U.S. children 6–17 years of age had current anxiety or depression that had previously been diagnosed by a healthcare provider. These parent-report data showed slightly more boys than girls had a diagnosis of anxiety or depression.

One in 24 children were diagnosed with anxiety in 2011–12, compared to the 2007 estimate of 1 in 28 children. Researchers also found that 1 in 37 children were diagnosed with depression in 2011–12, which is similar to the 2007 estimate.

Based on the 2011–12 data, children with current anxiety or depression were more likely than those without to have:
- Another mental, behavioral, or developmental disorder such as attention deficit hyperactivity disorder (ADHD), learning disability, or speech or language problems
- Other chronic health conditions, such as asthma or hearing problems
- School problems
- Parents who report high levels of stress and frustration with parenting
- Unmet medical and mental-health service needs

A large number of children and adolescents are diagnosed with anxiety and depression in the United States. It is important to monitor these conditions and how they are treated because they have a significant impact on overall health and relationships.

IMPACT OF MENTAL-HEALTH PROBLEMS IN ADOLESCENCE

It is a normal part of development for teens to experience a wide range of emotions. It is typical, for instance, for teens to feel anxious about school or friendships, or to experience a period of depression following the death of a close friend or family member. Mental-health disorders, however, are characterized by persistent symptoms that affect how a young person feels, thinks, and acts. Mental-health disorders also can interfere with regular activities and daily functioning, such as relationships, schoolwork, sleeping, and eating. When left untreated, mental-health disorders can lead to serious—even life-threatening—consequences. Depression, other mental-health disorders, and substance-use disorders are major risk factors for suicide. Suicide is the second leading cause of death for 15- to 24-year-olds. In 2013 and 2014, children ages 10 to 14 died from suicide than in a motor vehicle accident. Any concerns that family members or healthcare providers have about an adolescent's mental health should be promptly addressed.

Section 5.3 | Anxiety among Pregnant Women

This section includes text excerpted from "Moms-to-Be and Moms," *Eunice Kennedy Shriver* National Institute of Child Health and Human Development (NICHD), August 12, 2019.

Pregnancy and a new baby can bring a range of emotions. In fact, many women feel overwhelmed, sad, or anxious at different times during their pregnancy, and even after the baby is born. For many women, these feelings go away on their own. But, for some women, these emotions are more serious and may stay for some time.

These feelings are not something you caused by doing or not doing something. And, they can be treated if you seek help.

ARE YOU TALKING ABOUT POSTPARTUM DEPRESSION?

Postpartum depression is one name you might hear for depression and anxiety that can happen during and after pregnancy. But, it might not be the best way to describe what women feel.

The word "postpartum" means "after birth," so "postpartum depression" is talking only about depression after the baby is born.

For many women, this term is correct: they start feeling depressed sometime within the first year after they have the baby.

But, research shows that some women start to feel depression while they are still pregnant. You might hear the term "perinatal depression" to describe this situation. The word "perinatal" describes the time during pregnancy or just after birth.

It is now known that women may also experience anxiety around the time of pregnancy, beyond just being nervous about having a baby. Anxiety during and after pregnancy is as common as depression and may even happen at the same time as depression. So, you also may hear "perinatal depression and anxiety" or "perinatal mood and anxiety disorders" used to describe all of what women might feel.

No matter what you call them depression and anxiety that happen during pregnancy or after birth are real medical conditions, and they affect many women.

WHAT ARE SOME SIGNS OF DEPRESSION AND ANXIETY?

Women with depression or anxiety around pregnancy tell that they feel:

- Extremely sad or angry without warning
- Foggy or have trouble completing tasks
- "Robotic," like they are just going through the motions
- Very anxious around the baby and their other children
- Guilty and like they are failing at motherhood
- Unusually irritable or angry

They also often have:

- Little interest in things they used to enjoy
- Scary, upsetting thoughts that do not go away

HOW COMMON ARE DEPRESSION AND ANXIETY DURING PREGNANCY OR AFTER BIRTH?

Researchers believe that depression is one of the most common problems women experience during and after pregnancy. According to a national survey, about 1 in 8 women experience postpartum depression.

Anxiety during and after pregnancy is as common as depression and may happen at the same time as depression.

You may feel like you are the only person in the world who feels depressed and anxious during pregnancy or after your baby is born, but you are not alone.

WHAT ARE THE RISK FACTORS FOR DEPRESSION AND ANXIETY DURING PREGNANCY OR AFTER BIRTH?

Depression and anxiety during pregnancy or after birth can happen to anyone. However, several factors make some women more likely than others to experience one or both of these conditions. These risk factors include:

- A history of depression or anxiety, either during pregnancy or at other times
- Family history of depression or anxiety
- A difficult pregnancy or birth experience
- Giving birth to twins or other multiples
- Experiencing problems in your relationship with your partner
- Experiencing financial problems
- Receiving little or no support from family or friends to help you care for your baby
- Unplanned pregnancy

Although the causes of these conditions are not fully understood, researchers think depression and anxiety during this time may result from a mix of physical, emotional, and environmental factors.

CAN DEPRESSION AND ANXIETY DURING PREGNANCY OR AFTER BIRTH AFFECT YOUR BABY?

Yes—these medical conditions can affect your baby, but not directly. Early mother-child bonding is important for your baby's development and becoming close to your baby is a big part of that bonding. When you have depression or anxiety during pregnancy or after birth, it can be hard to become close to your baby. You may not be able to respond to what your baby needs. And, if there are older children in the house, they may be missing your support as well.

Early treatment is important for you, your baby, and the rest of your family. The sooner you start, the more quickly you will start to feel better.

Section 5.4 | Anxiety among Older Adults

This section includes text excerpted from "The State of Mental Health and Aging in America," Centers for Disease Control and Prevention (CDC), November 26, 2008. Reviewed August 2020.

MENTAL-HEALTH PROBLEMS IN OLDER ADULTS

It is estimated that 20 percent of people 55 years of age or older experience some type of mental-health concern. The most common conditions include anxiety, severe cognitive impairment, and mood disorders (such as depression or bipolar disorder). Mental-health issues are often implicated as a factor in cases of suicide. Older men have the highest suicide rate of any age group. Men 85 years of age or older have a suicide rate of 45.23 per 100,000, compared to an overall rate of 11.1 per 100,000 for all ages.

The Significance of Depression

Depression, a type of mood disorder, is the most prevalent mental-health problem among older adults. It is associated with distress and suffering. It also can lead to impairments in physical, mental, and social functioning. The presence of depressive disorders often adversely affects the course and complicates the treatment of other chronic diseases. Older adults with depression visit the doctor and emergency room more often, use more medication, incur higher outpatient charges, and stay longer in the hospital.

Although the rate of older adults with depressive symptoms tends to increase with age, depression is not a normal part of growing older. Rather, in 80 percent of cases, it is a treatable condition. Unfortunately, depressive disorders are a widely underrecognized condition and often are untreated or undertreated among older adults.

FREQUENT MENTAL DISTRESS

- Frequent mental distress (FMD) may interfere with major life activities such as eating well, maintaining a household, working, or sustaining personal relationships.
- FMD can also affect physical health. Older adults with FMD were more likely to engage in behaviors that can contribute to poor health, such as smoking, not getting recommended amounts of exercise, or eating a diet with few fruits and vegetables.
- The overwhelming majority of older adults did not experience FMD. In fact, in 2006, the prevalence of FMD was only 9.2 percent among U.S. adults 50 years of age or older and 6.5 percent among those 65 years of age or older.
- Hispanics had a higher prevalence of FMD (13.2%) compared to white, non-Hispanics (8.3%) or black, non-Hispanics (11.1%).
- Women 50 to 64 years of age and 65 or older reported more FMD than men in the same age groups (13.2% and 7.7% compared to 9.1% and 5%, respectively).

LIFETIME DIAGNOSIS OF ANXIETY DISORDER

- Anxiety, such as depression, is among the most prevalent mental-health problems among older adults. The two conditions often go hand in hand, with almost half of older adults who are diagnosed with major depression also meeting the criteria for anxiety.
- Late-life anxiety is not well-understood but is believed to be as common in older adults as in younger age groups (although how and when it appears is distinctly different in older adults). Anxiety in this age group may be underestimated because older adults are less likely to report psychiatric symptoms and more likely to emphasize physical complaints.

- More than 90 percent of adults 50 years of age or older did not report a lifetime diagnosis of anxiety.
- Adults 50 to 64 years of age reported a lifetime diagnosis of an existing anxiety disorder more than adults 65 years of age or older (12.7% compared to 7.6%).
- Hispanic adults 50 years of age or older were slightly more likely to report a lifetime diagnosis of an anxiety disorder compared to white, non-Hispanic, black, non-Hispanic, or other, non-Hispanic adults (14.5% compared to 12.6%, 11%, and 14.2%, respectively).
- Women 50 to 64 years of age report a lifetime diagnosis of an anxiety disorder more often than men in this age group (16.1% compared to 9.2%, respectively).

Section 5.5 | Anxiety among LGBTQ

"Anxiety among LGBTQ," © 2020 Omnigraphics. Reviewed August 2020.

There has been a substantial amount of public and scientific awareness in the past two decades about lesbian, gay, bisexual, transgender, and queer or questioning (LGBTQ) lives and the issues they face. This awareness began from more significant socio-cultural shifts in comprehending sexual and gender identities, such as the LGBT social movements in the 1970s. During recent times LGBTQ youth are known to "come out" at a younger age since public support and laws ruling in favor of the LGBTQ have considerably increased. However, LGBTQ people are still three times more likely to have a mental-health concern, when compared to straight people.

SOCIAL ANXIETY DISORDER IN LGBTQ

The LGBTQ individuals are often at an increased risk for social anxiety disorder (SAD) due to the social context in which they are forced to grow up. They may face stigma and prejudice for doing the same things that people take for granted, such as exhibiting a public display of affection. This creates the need to monitor oneself in social situations, leading to the development of SAD. About 30–60 percent of LGBTQ people are known to live with anxiety and depression at a certain point in their lives. They are also prone to be two times at higher risk for these disorders than other people. Some of the most common acts of discrimination and prejudice against members of the LGBTQ community that lead to anxiety disorders are:

- Constant threats to housing and employment opportunities
- Creating a need to hide their sexual identity in certain social situations
- Lack of family support
- Long-term effects of violence and bullying
- Low self-esteem

MINORITY STRESS

The process of dealing with persistent discrimination results in minority stress. It refers to chronic stress experienced by a group of people who experience stigma and prejudice, such as homophobia or transphobia. Studies show that minority stress has significant, lasting, and adverse influence on the mental health and well-being of LGBTQ people. It can also further the impact of struggling with anxiety disorder and depression. LGBTQ individuals may face subtle hints or blatant aggression to show that they are not approved if they "come out." This may force them to be silent about their sexual identity, resulting in increased levels of anxiety. A few other impacts of prejudicial treatment against the LGBTQ include:

- In 2017, about 40 percent of LGBTQ adults had a mental-health concern compared to 10 percent of the total adult population with mental-health problems.
- An estimated 20–30 percent of LGBTQ individuals are addicted to substance abuse, compared to 9 percent of the general population who abuse substances.
- A large number of LGBTQ people are ostracized by their families and asked to leave their homes.

According to the Trevor project survey, 71 percent of LGBTQ youth have been discriminated against due to their gender or sexual identity.

MENTAL-HEALTH SUPPORT FOR LGBTQ

In cases of severe anxiety, a doctor may prescribe medications to lower levels of anxiety and stress. However, medication is found to be most effective for social anxiety when combined with cognitive-behavioral therapy (CBT) or acceptance and commitment therapy (ACT). LGBTQ people require compassionate and informed mental-health support to survive the various forms of prejudice and discrimination they face in their daily lives. In the past few years, there have been considerable advances in the knowledge of policies and practices leading to the development of supportive school environments that have contributed to the positive mental health of LGBTQ youth. Meanwhile, mental-health support is seen to be lacking for most adults who are LGBTQ and some are even denied healthcare due to their sexual or gender identity.

References

1. "Mental Health in Lesbian, Gay, Bisexual, and Transgender (LGBT) Youth," National Center for Biotechnology Information, January 14, 2016.
2. Cuncic, Arlin. "Living with Social Anxiety Disorder as an LGBTQ+ Person," Verywell Mind, April 8, 2019.
3. O'Grady, Kevin. "Why Does the LGBT Community Experience Such High Levels of Anxiety?" Anxiety.org, June 26, 2015.
4. "LGBTQ+ Communities," Anxiety and Depression Association of America (ADAA), September 2, 2018.

Chapter 6 | **Quality of Life Impairments in Anxiety Disorder**

The quality of life (QOL) of a person is based on their perception of their position in life in relation to their standards, expectations, objectives, personal health, mental state, and concerns. It is also dependent on the culture and value systems in which a person lives. Individuals with generalized anxiety disorder (GAD), including social phobia and panic disorder are known to have less satisfaction with their quality of life than other nonanxious adults. Anxiety disorder causes people to live in constant and often unbiased fear, limiting them from trying new things in personal life and work or even making it hard for them to step out of the house. This can also eventually lead to poor physical and mental health.

IMPACT OF ANXIETY DISORDER ON SCHOOL LIFE

Anxiety disorder (AD) has a significant impact on academic performance, classroom behavior, and social interactions of students. According to the Anxiety and Depression Association of America (ADAA), 1 in every 8 children has anxiety; 80 percent children with anxiety disorder and 60 percent of children with depression are not receiving treatment. The following are some of the significant implications of AD on students:

"Quality of Life Impairments in Anxiety Disorder," © 2020 Omnigraphics. Reviewed August 2020.

1. **Difficulty in paying attention.** Excessive anxiety causes students to worry about several things at once, which hinders their ability to focus on class and follow complicated instructions.
2. **Unable to process information.** Sometimes anxious students do pay attention in class; however, their cognitive abilities are taken over by anxiety and the information is only processed on a surface-level. This also incapacitates their ability to multitask or do complex projects.
3. **Inability to use long-term memory.** Since the information is not processed properly, students have trouble accessing it from long-term memory, where informative knowledge is stored indefinitely. This leads to students developing "test anxiety," which further reduces the ability to access the information.

Despite these issues, it is still possible for students with anxiety disorders to perform well similar to nonanxious students. However, it requires way more effort, and a considerable amount of stress builds up over a period of time. It is necessary for teachers to focus on and evaluate the student's work patterns and methods, along with their grades. Identifying academic, social, or behavioral challenges sooner can help teachers work better with the students and their parents to address anxiety disorders, so that the student's performance is not affected.

IMPACT OF ANXIETY DISORDER ON JOB PERFORMANCE

Work-related anxiety can result from excessive demands, toxic work culture, unhealthy work pressure, and a poorly matched job description. The symptoms of anxiety disorder can manifest differently in a workplace and affect several areas of work-life. A few common effects of workplace anxiety are:

- Difficulty working with clients and colleagues
- Trouble focusing on the assigned task
- Being preoccupied with unbiased fear
- Refusing assignments due to fear of failure

- Using stairs to avoid risking conversation in elevators
- Turning down opportunities due to fear of public speaking

It is important to try tackling these issues by seeking help from a therapist or talking about it with your employer or supportive coworkers. Additionally, relaxation techniques, including deep breathing, may help ease muscle tension and other physical symptoms caused due to anxiety. However, if the job is proving to be a constant source of stress and excessive anxiety, changing work positions or changing the job entirely would be the only other option.

IMPACT OF ANXIETY DISORDER ON PERSONAL RELATIONSHIPS

Depending on the symptoms experienced, anxiety disorders can impact the personal relationships of a person in many different ways:

- **Dependence.** Anxiety can sometimes make a person overly dependent on their partner. This is usually caused due to nervousness to face a situation alone, fear of rejection, and being indecisive, making them crave constant reassurance and support from their loved ones. This can also lead to overthinking when a person does not respond quickly via social media or phone. They may often face trouble with effective communication and act in a destructive way that might cause their loved ones to maintain physical and emotional distance.
- **Isolation.** Others with anxiety may choose to socially isolate themselves and avoid relationships to protect themselves from feeling unfavorable emotions such as being disappointed or frustrated with a loved one. This results in having difficulty opening up or being vulnerable with loved ones, which makes them seem cold, indifferent, and emotionally unavailable.

Therapists can help people explore how anxiety disorders are impacting a relationship. For example, deeply exploring emotions might help individuals who tend to avoid relationships to express themselves better. Similarly, cognitive-behavioral therapy (CBT), enables a person to recognize and alter their thought patterns and behaviors that cause anxious feelings. This can be beneficial for overdependent people as it helps them reduce distorted thinking by enabling them to look at concerns more realistically.

IMPACTS OF ANXIETY ON SOCIAL RELATIONSHIPS

About 15 million American adults are affected by social anxiety disorder (SAD), the second most common anxiety disorder after specific phobia. SAD, also known as "social phobia," is characterized by an intense fear of being judged, negative criticism, or rejected in a social situation. It often causes people to be extremely concerned about appearing visibly anxious (blushing or stammering) or being viewed as awkward, clumsy, and annoying. Due to this, they often avoid social circumstances and might have difficulty understanding how others manage so easily in such situations. However, avoiding most social situations not only affects relationships but can also result in developing:

1. Negative thoughts/feelings
2. Low self-confidence
3. Sensitivity to criticism
4. Mental depression
5. Difficulty being assertive

People diagnosed with SAD are often at an increased risk of developing alcohol-use disorders and major depressive disorders. There are numerous effective treatments available to treat SADs, but less than 5 percent of people with SAD get treated a year after the symptoms begin to manifest. Most others live with the symptoms for more than 10 years before finally seeking treatment.

Medications are considered a vital part of treating anxiety disorders, especially for people whose daily functioning is affected due to anxiety. Medications prescribed for anxiety include serotonin-norepinephrine reuptake inhibitors (SNRIs) and selective serotonin reuptake inhibitors (SSRIs). These medications cannot completely cure anxiety, but they help reduce the symptoms and assist people in working through their anxious emotions and behaviors with a therapist. Anxiety disorders are usually persistent and last a lifetime, which can result in a considerable impairment in the quality of life for both the patient and their families.

References

1. Meek, William. "How Anxiety May Affect Your Relationships," Very Well Mind, March 25, 2020.
2. "Social Anxiety Disorder," Anxiety and Depression Association of America (ADAA), October 20, 2017.
3. "Impact of Anxiety/OCD at School," Anxiety in the Classroom, September 30, 2018.
4. Cuncic, Arlin. "An Overview of Work Anxiety," Very Well Mind, March 22, 2020.
5. "Quality of Life Impairment in Depression and Anxiety Disorders," Medical Journal of D.Y. Patil Vidyapeeth, July 5, 2013.

Chapter 7 | **Prevalence of Anxiety Disorders in the United States**

The wide variety of anxiety disorders differ by the objects or situations that induce them, but share features of excessive anxiety and related behavioral disturbances. Anxiety disorders can interfere with daily activities such as job performance, school work, and relationships.

PREVALENCE OF ANY ANXIETY DISORDER AMONG ADULTS

- Based on diagnostic interview data from the National Comorbidity Study Replication (NCS-R), figure 7.1. shows the past-year prevalence of any anxiety disorder among U.S. adults 18 years of age or older.
  - An estimated 19.1 percent of U.S. adults had any anxiety disorder in the past year.
  - Past year prevalence of any anxiety disorder was higher for females (23.4%) than for males (14.3%).
- An estimated 31.1 percent of U.S. adults experience any anxiety disorder at some time in their lives.

ANY ANXIETY DISORDER WITH IMPAIRMENT AMONG ADULTS

- Of adults with any anxiety disorder in the past year, the degree of impairment ranged from mild-to-severe, as

This chapter includes text excerpted from "Any Anxiety Disorder," National Institute of Mental Health (NIMH), November 2017.

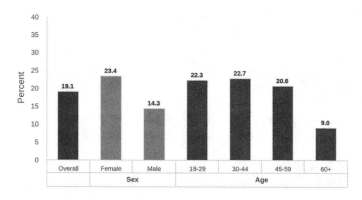

Figure 7.1. Past Year Prevalence of Any Anxiety Disorder among U.S. Adult (2001–2003)

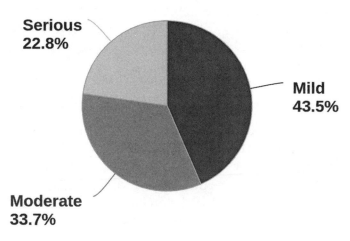

Figure 7.2. Past Year Severity of Any Anxiety Disorder among U.S. Adult (2001–2003)

shown in figure 7.2. Impairment was determined by scores on the Sheehan Disability Scale (SDS).

- Among adults with any anxiety disorder, an estimated 22.8 percent had serious impairment, and 33.7 percent had moderate impairment.
- A majority of people with any anxiety disorder experienced mild impairment (43.5%).

Prevalence of Anxiety Disorders in the United States

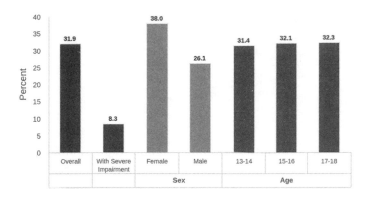

Figure 7.3. Lifetime Prevalence of Any Anxiety Disorder among Adolescents (2001–2004)

PREVALENCE OF ANY ANXIETY DISORDER AMONG ADOLESCENTS

- Based on diagnostic interview data from the National Comorbidity Survey Adolescent Supplement (NCS-A), figure 7.3. shows the lifetime prevalence of any anxiety disorder among U.S. adolescents 13 to 18 years of age.
  - An estimated 31.9 percent of adolescents had any anxiety disorder.
  - Of adolescents with any anxiety disorder, an estimated 8.3 percent had severe impairment. DSM-IV criteria were used to determine impairment.
  - The prevalence of any anxiety disorder among adolescents was higher for females (38.0%) than for males (26.1%).
  - The prevalence of any anxiety disorder was similar across age groups.

Part 2 | Types of Anxiety Disorders

Chapter 8 | Generalized Anxiety Disorder

WHAT IS GENERALIZED ANXIETY DISORDER?[1]

Occasional anxiety is a normal part of life. You might worry about things such as health, money, or family problems. But, people with generalized anxiety disorder (GAD) feel extremely worried or feel nervous about these and other things—even when there are little or no reasons to worry about them. People with GAD find it difficult to control their anxiety and stay focused on daily tasks. The good news is that GAD is treatable. Call your doctor to talk about your symptoms so that you can feel better.

WHAT ARE THE SIGNS AND SYMPTOMS OF GENERALIZED ANXIETY DISORDER?[1]

Generalized anxiety disorder develops slowly. It often starts during the teen years or young adulthood. People with GAD may:
- Worry very much about everyday things
- Have trouble controlling their worries or feelings of nervousness
- Know that they worry much more than they should
- Feel restless and have trouble relaxing
- Have a hard time concentrating
- Be easily startled
- Have trouble falling asleep or staying asleep

This chapter includes text excerpted from documents published by two public domain sources. Text under the headings marked 1 are excerpted from "Generalized Anxiety Disorder: When Worry Gets Out of Control," National Institute of Mental Health (NIMH), 2016. Reviewed August 2020; Text under the headings marked 2 are excerpted from "What Is Generalized Anxiety Disorder," Mental Illness Research, Education and Clinical Centers (MIRECC), U.S. Department of Veterans Affairs (VA), 2019.

- Feel easily tired or tired all the time
- Have headaches, muscle aches, stomach aches, or unexplained pains
- Have a hard time swallowing
- Tremble or twitch
- Be irritable or feel "on edge"
- Sweat a lot, feel light-headed or out of breath
- Have to go to the bathroom a lot

Children and teens with GAD often worry excessively about:
- Their performance, such as in school or in sports
- Catastrophes, such as earthquakes or war

Adults with GAD are often highly nervous about everyday circumstances, such as:
- Job security or performance
- Health
- Finances
- The health and well-being of their children
- Being late
- Completing household chores and other responsibilities

Both children and adults with GAD may experience physical symptoms that make it hard to function and that interfere with daily life.

PREVALENCE[2]

Approximately 5.7 percent of people will have a diagnosis of GAD at some point in their lifetime, and it is about twice as common in females. Subclinical GAD is even more common than GAD. This is defined as having some symptoms of the disorder, but not enough for a diagnosis to be made. An additional 8 to 13.7 percent of people will experience subclinical GAD at some point in their life. Even though they do not have all the symptoms needed for a diagnosis of GAD, they too have higher levels of distress and impairment in their lives as compared to those without these anxiety symptoms.

They are also at risk for developing another psychiatric disorder; between 42 to 86.3 percent of those with subclinical GAD have symptoms or a diagnosis of another disorder.

WHAT CAUSES GENERALIZED ANXIETY DISORDER[1]

Generalized anxiety disorder sometimes runs in families, but no one knows for sure why some family members have it while others do not. Researchers have found that several parts of the brain, as well as biological processes, play a key role in fear and anxiety. By learning more about how the brain and body function in people with anxiety disorders, researchers may be able to create better treatments. Researchers are also looking for ways in which stress and environmental factors play a role.

HOW FAMILY MEMBERS CAN HELP[2]
Encourage Treatment

Generalized anxiety disorder is a treatable problem. Psychotherapy and medications can help ease the symptoms of GAD and reduce distress. It is important for a person with GAD to first visit a mental-health professional for a thorough evaluation. If possible, family members could also attend to help answer questions and to provide support. If the person with GAD is prescribed medications that need to be taken at regular times, the family member can help give support around that. Taking medication can be difficult—there might be times when a person does not want to take it or just might forget to take it. Family members can help encourage and remind them to take their medications. Family members can also support attendance to psychotherapy appointments by giving reminders and providing transportation.

Reinforce Treatment Concepts

Generalized anxiety disorder can have a negative impact on the family. For example, family members might be pulled into providing reassurance for anxious thoughts. Although family members might feel like they are "helping" their relative by providing reassurance, these behaviors actually make things worse. Reassurance reinforces worries and anxiety. The affected family member can become dependent on the reassurance. As a result, they do not learn how to tolerate anxiety and uncertainty, and things do not get better. How can family members eliminate providing reassurance? For example, when asked by their relative with GAD for reassurance, family members can gently say something like, "I cannot answer that for you, see if you can sit with these feelings."

Family members often feel guilty about not providing reassurance but having an understanding of the cognitive-behavioral model of GAD can help reduce feelings of guilt. Family members can talk with a CBT therapist to learn specifics about how they can reduce providing reassurance and provide support for the treatment. For example, CBT is comprised of homework assignments; family members can encourage their relatives to engage in the homework such as cognitive restructuring, and offer to help, if relevant. If mindfulness is part of the treatment, family members can offer to join in such practice at home. If the family member with GAD is dealing with insomnia, family members can help by supporting positive sleep behaviors (e.g., not working or using electronics in bed themselves and not bringing up challenging discussion topics right before bed). Even if a person is not receiving psychotherapy for GAD, relatives can help reinforce some of these concepts.

Take Care of Themselves

Given some of the challenges that family members may face, it is important that they take care of themselves as well. There are many ways to do this. Family members should not allow their relatives with GAD to monopolize all of their time, and spending time alone or with other family members or friends is important for their own well-being. Family members may also consider joining a support or therapy group. Counseling can often help family and friends better cope with a loved one's GAD. Finally, family members should not feel responsible for solving the problem themselves. They cannot. They should get the help of a mental-health professional if needed.

Chapter 9 | **Separation Anxiety Disorder**

WHAT IS SEPARATION ANXIETY DISORDER?

Individuals with separation anxiety disorder (SAD) worry excessively when they anticipate or experience separation from parents or loved ones. Children with SAD experience extreme distress when they are away from parents or caregivers and fear they could get lost from their family or think something bad is happening to their family while they are apart. Separation anxiety is normal in early childhood, but it becomes a disorder when anxiety interferes with age-appropriate activities and behavior. SAD is most often diagnosed in children during preschool and the early school years, but in rare cases, it can become a problem in early adolescence. It is estimated that about 4 percent of all children have this disorder, which can be treated with behavioral and pharmacological therapy if identified early.

WHAT ARE THE CHARACTERISTICS OF SEPARATION ANXIETY DISORDER?

Symptoms exhibited with SAD tend to vary with each individual, but some common characteristics include:

- Overattachment to parents or loved ones and a perception of danger to family during separation
- Worry and stress before or during separation from parents or loved ones
- Complaints of headache, nausea, dizziness, or other physical symptoms when separation is anticipated

"Separation Anxiety Disorder," © 2018 Omnigraphics. Reviewed August 2020.

- Having a hard time saying goodbye to parents, throwing tantrums when faced with separation, feeling afraid of staying alone in one part of a house, or fear of sleeping in a darkened room
- Being afraid of staying home in the absence of parents or loved ones
- Worrisome thoughts of harm to parents or loved ones (e.g., accident, illness, or death)
- Persistent thoughts of the dangers of being separated from loved ones, such as being kidnapped or getting lost
- An overwhelming need to know where parents are when apart, often phoning or texting
- Difficulty falling asleep away from home
- Nightmares with themes of separation from parents or loved ones
- Avoiding playtime, birthday parties, and other activities away from loved ones
- Obsessively shadowing a parent at home or elsewhere
- Refusal to leave home or go to school

WHAT CAUSES SEPARATION ANXIETY DISORDER

Biological and environmental factors could all contribute to SAD. Other causes can include chemical imbalances, possibly of such substances as norepinephrine and serotonin in the brain. There could be a biological tendency to feel anxious, but the disorder could also be the result of behavior learned from family members who display elevated anxiety levels around the child. It is also possible that SAD could result from a traumatic childhood experience.

WHO IS AFFECTED BY SEPARATION ANXIETY DISORDER?

A certain degree of separation anxiety is normal in children, and dealing with it is a natural part of growing up. SAD is identified when anxiety about being apart from home and family is far beyond that of typical child development. It occurs equally in both sexes, and symptoms usually surface in children following a break from school, such as after Christmas vacation or a period of extended illness. Children of parents with this disorder have a higher than average likelihood of developing the same condition.

HOW IS SEPARATION ANXIETY DISORDER DIAGNOSED?

A child psychiatrist or other mental-health professional diagnoses SAD on the basis of a psychological evaluation. Diagnosis involves identifying and quantifying the distress experienced by the individual during separation from parents or loved ones. Among other factors, the child must experience the symptoms for at least four weeks to meet the technical criteria for SAD. A clinician will be able to determine if the symptoms are otherwise only a temporary response to a stressful life situation.

WHAT IS THE TREATMENT FOR SEPARATION ANXIETY DISORDER?

The diagnostician will evaluate the condition of the child and decide on treatment based on the severity of symptoms, age of the child, health and medical history, tolerance for medication and therapy, and personal preference for mode of treatment. The first line of treatment in SAD is psychotherapy. Cognitive-behavioral therapy (CBT), in particular, has been very successful in mild-to-moderate cases.

The focus of treatment is to provide the child with the skills to manage anxiety and master the situations that contribute to the symptoms of SAD. Exposure therapy, a modified version of CBT is recommended in certain cases. Here, the child is exposed to separation in small, controlled doses, which helps reduce anxiety gradually over time. In severe cases that do not respond to psychotherapy, medication may be required. In such cases, selective serotonin reuptake inhibitors (SSRIs), antidepressants, and antianxiety medications are often prescribed to make the child feel calmer.

HOW IS SEPARATION ANXIETY DISORDER PREVENTED?

Preventive measures are presently unknown. Instead of prevention, the focus is on early detection and intervention, which can successfully reduce the severity of the disorder and enhance normal growth and development patterns, while improving the quality of life for affected children.

References

1. "Separation Anxiety Disorder," Jane and Terry Semel Institute for Neuroscience and Human Behavior, n.d.
2. "Separation Anxiety Disorder," Stanford Children's Health, n.d.
3. "Separation Anxiety Disorder," Child Mind Institute, n.d.

Chapter 10 | **Specific Phobias**

A phobia is a type of anxiety disorder. It is a strong, irrational fear of something that poses little or no actual danger. There are many specific phobias. Acrophobia is a fear of heights. You may be able to ski the world's tallest mountains but be unable to go above the 5th floor of an office building. Agoraphobia is a fear of public places, and claustrophobia is a fear of closed-in places. If you become anxious and extremely self-conscious in everyday social situations, you could have a social phobia. Other common phobias involve tunnels, highway driving, water, flying, animals, and blood.

People with phobias try to avoid what they are afraid of. If they cannot, they may experience:
- Panic and fear
- Rapid heartbeat
- Shortness of breath
- Trembling
- A strong desire to get away

Treatment helps most people with phobias. Options include medicines, therapy, or both.

This chapter contains text excerpted from the following sources: Text in this chapter begins with excerpts from "Phobias," MentalHealth.gov, U.S. Department of Health and Human Services (HHS), August 22, 2017; Text under the heading "What Is Specific Phobias?" is excerpted from "Specific Phobias," U.S. Department of Veterans Affairs (VA), December 23, 2019; Text beginning with the heading "Prevalence of Specific Phobia among Adults" is excerpted from "Specific Phobias," National Institute of Mental Health (NIMH), November 2017.

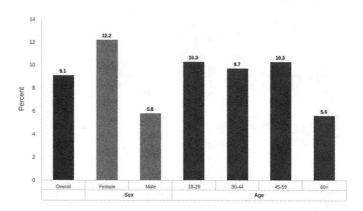

Figure 10.1. Past Year Prevalence of Specific Phobia among Adults

WHAT IS SPECIFIC PHOBIA?

As the name suggests, a person with a specific phobia experiences intense fear in response to an object or situation. For example, fear of blood or needles, fear of enclosed places, and fear of flying are common specific phobias, with fear of spiders, fear of snakes, and fear of heights being most common. While many people describe being very afraid of certain situations or things, they may not be bothered by their fear or it may not stop them from doing things because they do not worry about being faced with the feared situation or object. For example, for a man who lives in New York City, a fear of snakes may not be very concerning to him and it likely does not get in the way of him doing things he needs to do. In this case, the fear would not necessarily be considered a specific phobia and he probably would not have a need for treatment.

PREVALENCE OF SPECIFIC PHOBIA AMONG ADULTS

- Based on diagnostic interview data from the National Comorbidity Survey Replication (NCS-R), figure 10.1. shows past-year prevalence of specific phobia among U.S. adults 18 years of age or older.
  - An estimated 9.1 percent of U.S. adults had specific phobia in the past year.

Specific Phobias

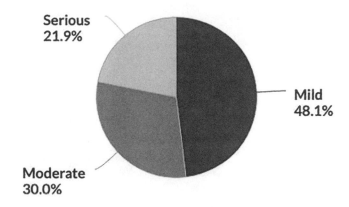

Figure 10.2. Past Year Severity of Specific Phobia with Impairment among Adults (2001–2003)

- Past year prevalence of specific phobia among adults was higher for females (12.2%) than for males (5.8%).
- An estimated 12.5 percent of U.S. adults experience specific phobia at some time in their lives.

SPECIFIC PHOBIA WITH IMPAIRMENT AMONG ADULTS

Of adults with specific phobia in the past year, degree of impairment ranged from mild-to-serious, as shown in Figure 10.2. Impairment was determined by scores on the Sheehan Disability Scale (SDS).

Of adults with specific phobia in the past year, an estimated 21.9 percent had serious impairment, 30.0 percent had moderate impairment, and 48.1 percent had mild impairment.

LIFETIME PREVALENCE OF SPECIFIC PHOBIA AMONG ADOLESCENTS

- Based on diagnostic interview data from the National Comorbidity Survey Adolescent Supplement (NCS-A), Figure 10.3. shows lifetime prevalence of specific phobia among U.S. adolescents 13 to 18 years of age.
- An estimated 19.3 percent of adolescents had specific phobia, and an estimated 0.6 percent had severe

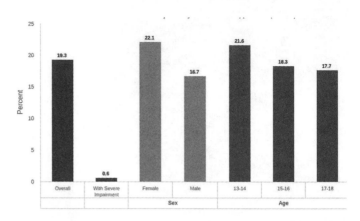

Figure 10.3. Lifetime Prevalence of Specific Phobia among Adolescents

impairment. *Diagnostic and Statistical Manual of Mental Disorders, Fourth Edition* (DSM-IV) criteria were used to determine impairment.

- The prevalence of specific phobia among adolescents was higher for females (22.1%) than for males (16.7%).

Chapter 11 | Social Anxiety Disorder (Social Phobia)

Are you extremely afraid of being judged by others? Are you very self-conscious in everyday social situations? Do you avoid meeting new people?

If you have been feeling this way for at least six months and these feelings make it hard for you to do everyday tasks—such as talking to people at work or school—you may have a social anxiety disorder.

Social anxiety disorder (also called "social phobia") is a mental-health condition. It is an intense, persistent fear of being watched and judged by others. This fear can affect work, school, and other day-to-day activities. It can even make it hard to make and keep friends. But, social anxiety disorder does not have to stop you from reaching your potential. Treatment can help you overcome your symptoms.

WHAT IS SOCIAL ANXIETY DISORDER?

Social anxiety disorder is a common type of anxiety disorder. A person with social anxiety disorder feels symptoms of anxiety or fear in certain, or all social situations such as meeting new people, dating, being on a job interview, answering a question in class, or having to talk to a cashier in a store. Doing everyday things in front of people—such as eating or drinking in front of others or using a public restroom—also causes anxiety or fear. The person is afraid that she or he will be humiliated, judged, and rejected.

This chapter includes text excerpted from "Social Anxiety Disorder: More than Just Shyness," National Institute of Mental Health (NIMH), December 21, 2016. Reviewed August 2020.

The fear that people with social anxiety disorder have in social situations is so strong that they feel it is beyond their ability to control. As a result, it gets in the way of going to work, attending school, or doing everyday things. People with social anxiety disorder may worry about these and other things for weeks before they happen. Sometimes, they end up staying away from places or events where they think they might have to do something that will embarrass them.

Some people with the disorder do not have anxiety in social situations but have performance anxiety instead. They feel physical symptoms of anxiety in situations such as giving a speech, playing a sports game, or dancing or playing a musical instrument on stage.

Social anxiety disorder usually starts during youth in people who are extremely shy. Social anxiety disorder is not uncommon; research suggests that about 7 percent of Americans are affected. Without treatment, social anxiety disorder can last for many years or a lifetime and prevent a person from reaching her or his full potential.

WHAT ARE THE SIGNS AND SYMPTOMS OF SOCIAL ANXIETY DISORDER?

When having to perform in front of or be around others, people with social anxiety disorder tend to:

- Blush, sweat, tremble, feel a rapid heart rate, or feel their "mind going blank"
- Feel nauseous or sick to their stomach
- Show a rigid body posture, make little eye contact, or speak with an overly soft voice
- Find it scary and difficult to be with other people, especially those they do not already know, and have a hard time talking to them even though they wish they could
- Be very self-conscious in front of other people and feel embarrassed and awkward
- Be very afraid that other people will judge them
- Stay away from places where there are other people

WHAT CAUSES SOCIAL ANXIETY DISORDER

Social anxiety disorder sometimes runs in families, but no one knows for sure why some family members have it while others do not. Researchers have found that several parts of the brain are involved in fear and anxiety. Some researchers think that the misreading of others' behavior may play a role in causing or worsening social anxiety. For example, you may think that people are staring or frowning at you when they truly are not. Underdeveloped social skills are another possible contributor to social anxiety. For example, if you have underdeveloped social skills, you may feel discouraged after talking with people and may worry about doing it in the future. By learning more about fear and anxiety in the brain, scientists may be able to create better treatments. Researchers are also looking for ways in which stress and environmental factors may play a role.

Chapter 12 | Selective Mutism

WHAT IS SELECTIVE MUTISM?

Selective mutism (SM) is a social anxiety disorder that is most often seen in children. Individuals with SM are unable to speak in certain social settings and with certain people. A child with SM may speak normally with parents and a few others but have difficulty speaking, or speaking above a whisper, in specific settings, such as school, public places, or family gatherings. The condition is quite rare, with fewer than 1 percent of cases documented in school, clinical, and child-guidance casework.

Children with SM typically fail to talk in school, which can interfere with academic and social performance. They sometimes communicate nonverbally by nodding, pointing, or writing, but some children remain motionless and expressionless until others correctly guess what they need. SM can cause considerable distress in certain instances, such as when the child does not communicate in times of pain or when needing to use the bathroom.

Children with SM possess the desire to speak but hold back because of anxiety, embarrassment, and shyness. It is important to understand that the child does not willfully refuse to speak but rather is unable to do so in particular situations. As a result, they often fail to participate in age-appropriate activities in and outside of school. SM is not to be confused with such behavior as shyness during the first few weeks of school or reticence to speak when a child is adapting to a new language.

WHAT ARE THE SIGNS AND SYMPTOMS OF SELECTIVE MUTISM?

The diagnostic criteria laid down in the *Diagnostic and Statistical Manual of Mental Disorders, 5th Edition* (DSM-5) include:

- Consistent failure to talk in social situations in which the child is expected to speak—in school, for example—despite speaking in other situations
- The inability to talk interferes with educational and occupational achievements or social interaction
- The problem lasts for at least one month in duration but is not limited to the first month in school
- The failure to speak in social situations cannot be attributed to lack of knowledge or comfort with using language
- The condition cannot be explained by communication disorders or mental-health issues, such as autism or schizophrenia

Children with SM may also display symptoms related to social anxiety and social phobia, such as:

- Being overly attached to parents
- Hiding, running away, freezing, and crying
- Being traumatized when asked to respond verbally in public
- Becoming anxious when a picture or video is taken
- Avoiding eating in public
- Being anxious about using public restrooms

Children with SM avoid conversations in many situations, and if they are able to express themselves, frequently do so by gesturing, nodding, and pointing. They often fear being ignored, ridiculed, or harshly evaluated if they try to speak.

WHAT ARE THE CAUSES AND RISK FACTORS OF SELECTIVE MUTISM?

The causes of SM are not yet definitively known, but multiple factors may play a role. For example, some research studies point to genetic influence as a possible cause for a predisposition to the condition. In many cases, it has been found that parents or other family members currently or previously have had symptoms related to extreme shyness, panic attacks, and social anxiety.

Some of the risk factors associated with SM include extreme shyness, a family history of the condition, or an anxiety disorder, such as panic disorder, or obsessive-compulsive behavior. In addition, research has shown that SM is four times more common in immigrant children than in the general population.

HOW IS SELECTIVE MUTISM DIAGNOSED?

Diagnosis of SM is based on the crucial observation that the child can comprehend language and speak normally but consistently fails to do so in specific settings. For instance, the child typically displays appropriate verbal skills at home with parents and certain other individuals with whom they are comfortable. In order to arrive at a diagnosis, a doctor or mental-health professional will rely on reports from parents and other adults who are in contact with the child to determine patterns across a variety of situations. Sometimes the diagnostician may ask for videos of the child in places where she or he is able to speak normally.

Specifically, the diagnosis is based on the child having the ability to speak in some settings and not in others, and in particular it must not relate to such temporary situations as the first month of school. For the diagnosis to be confirmed, the inability to speak must interfere with schooling and other social activities that most children are otherwise able to negotiate easily.

HOW IS SELECTIVE MUTISM TREATED?

Early intervention is crucial for the successful treatment of SM. The most effective treatment has been shown to be behavioral therapy using controlled exposure. The therapist works with the child and parents and systematically approaches the settings in which the child cannot speak. The therapist gradually builds the child's confidence, one situation at a time, during which she or he is never pressured to speak. Instead, the child is encouraged with positive reinforcement. The therapist provides the parents with specialized techniques to apply in real-life settings. The predictability and control that therapy gives the child helps reduce anxiety and improves self-image as a result of the mastery of speaking skills in various settings.

Medication may be prescribed, but this is not required in all cases of SM. However, if conditions are severe, a physician may prescribe antianxiety medications. In addition, a history of similar disorders in the family and lack of response to behavioral therapy and other forms of psychotherapy may prompt the need for pharmacological intervention. In many cases, when medication has been prescribed, children are better able to deal with exposure tasks in behavior therapy, which can help lead to successful treatment. The classes of medications prescribed for SM include selective serotonin reuptake inhibitors (SSRIs) and other antidepressants. Some children respond well to SSRIs in the case of anxiety, but they need to be monitored carefully for side effects.

WHAT ARE OTHER CONCERNS RELATED TO SELECTIVE MUTISM?

At one time, a common theory held that SM was often closely related to child abuse, but according to the Selective Mutism Foundation, research has since discarded this line of thinking. The suggestion of child abuse is devastating to families, and it has deterred many parents from seeking appropriate help for their child's SM. Child abuse can cause similar symptoms in children, but it may not be specific to immediate family members and could be due to other adults or even children. It is best to contact appropriate agencies in suspected cases of child abuse.

Selective Mutism is sometimes mistaken for autism, since many children with this disorder also experience speech and language problems. The crucial difference is that children with SM have the ability to speak and function normally in some settings.

Selective Mutism is not necessarily limited to children. Most children who experience SM at a young age do so for a short period, but others may find that it continues over many years. If misdiagnosed or improperly treated, SM could persist into adulthood. Studies have shown that some adults report struggling with the symptoms of SM and having to deal with residual symptoms, such as shyness, social anxiety, depression, and panic attacks for many years.

Parents can help children with SM by providing them with opportunities to socialize and speak in low-stress settings. They can implement behavioral techniques in all social situations in which the child finds it difficult to speak. To do this properly, parents should enlist the assistance of school authorities, teachers, school psychologists, guidance counsellors, and social workers to implement a consistent treatment plan.

References

1. "Selective Mutism (SM) Basics," Child Mind Institute, n.d.
2. "Understanding Selective Mutism Brochure. A Silent Cry for Help!" Selective Mutism Foundation, n.d.
3. "Selective Mutism," The American Speech-Language-Hearing Association (ASHA), n.d.

Chapter 13 | **Panic Disorders**

Do you sometimes have sudden attacks of anxiety and overwhelming fear that last for several minutes? Maybe your heart pounds, you sweat, and you feel like you cannot breathe or think. Do these attacks occur at unpredictable times with no obvious trigger, causing you to worry about the possibility of having another one at any time?

If so, you may have a type of anxiety disorder called "panic disorder." Left untreated, panic disorder can lower your quality of life (QOL) because it may lead to other fears and mental-health disorders, problems at work or school, and social isolation.

WHAT IS PANIC DISORDER?

People with panic disorder have sudden and repeated attacks of fear that last for several minutes or longer. These are called "panic attacks." Panic attacks are characterized by a fear of disaster or of losing control even when there is no real danger. A person may also have a strong physical reaction during a panic attack. It may feel like having a heart attack.

A person with panic disorder may become discouraged and feel ashamed because she or he cannot carry out normal routines such as going to school or work, going to the grocery store, or driving.

Panic disorder often begins in the late teens or early adulthood. More women than men have panic disorder. But, not everyone who experiences panic attacks will develop panic disorder.

This chapter includes text excerpted from "Panic Disorder: When Fear Overwhelms," National Institute of Mental Health (NIMH), 2016. Reviewed August 2020.

WHAT CAUSES PANIC DISORDER

Panic disorder sometimes runs in families, but no one knows for sure why some family members have it while others do not. Researchers have found that several parts of the brain, as well as biological processes, play a key role in fear and anxiety. Some researchers think that people with panic disorder misinterpret harmless bodily sensations as threats. By learning more about how the brain and body function in people with panic disorder, scientists may be able to create better treatments. Researchers are also looking for ways in which stress and environmental factors may play a role.

WHAT ARE THE SIGNS AND SYMPTOMS OF PANIC DISORDER?

People with panic disorder may have:

- Sudden and repeated panic attacks of overwhelming anxiety and fear
- A feeling of being out of control, or a fear of death or impending doom during a panic attack
- Physical symptoms during a panic attack such as a pounding or racing heart, sweating, chills, trembling, breathing problems, weakness or dizziness, tingly or numb hands, chest pain, stomach pain, and nausea
- An intense worry about when the next panic attack will happen
- A fear or avoidance of places where panic attacks have occurred in the past

Chapter 14 | **Agoraphobia**

The word agoraphobia literally means "fear of wide, open spaces." However, people with a diagnosis of agoraphobia might also have extreme fear or anxiety of other types of situations, such as being out of their home alone or being in a crowd. Individuals with agoraphobia often try to avoid these feared situations because of their high levels of anxiety. If avoidance is not possible, they need to be accompanied by another person, and/or they endure the situations with extreme anxiety. These situations are often avoided for fear of having a panic attack. Thus many people with a diagnosis of agoraphobia also have a diagnosis of panic disorder.

RISK FACTORS OF AGORAPHOBIA
The risk factors for agoraphobia are very similar for those described for panic disorder, and it is likely that genetic, biological, personality, and environmental stressors all play a role in the development of the disorder. For those who develop agoraphobia after having panic attacks, the stated cause of avoidance of certain situations is usually a fear of panicking in those situations.

DIAGNOSIS OF AGORAPHOBIA
To receive a diagnosis of agoraphobia, a person needs to exhibit high levels of fear or anxiety about at least two of the following situations, for at least six months or longer:
- Using public transportation

This chapter contains text excerpted from the following sources: Text in this chapter begins with excerpts from "What Are Panic Disorder and Agoraphobia," Mental Illness Research, Education and Clinical Centers (MIRECC), U.S. Department of Veterans Affairs (VA), 2016. Reviewed August 2020; Text under the heading "Prevalence of Agoraphobia among Adults" is excerpted from "Agoraphobia," National Institute of Mental Health (NIMH), November 2017.

- Being in open spaces, such as parks or on bridges
- Being in enclosed places such as theaters or stores
- Being in a crowd or standing in line
- Being outside of the home alone

A person with a diagnosis of agoraphobia fears or avoids these situations because they are concerned that they will not be able to escape them. Others fear that they might not receive help if they develop panic-like symptoms or other incapacitating or embarrassing symptoms (such as fear of incontinence or fear of falling in the elderly). The situations almost always cause fear or anxiety in the individuals with agoraphobia, and their fears are out of proportion with the actual danger involved in approaching these situations. The fear or avoidance must cause significant distress or impairment in major areas of functioning in order to receive a diagnosis of agoraphobia. If a person is avoiding these situations because of concerns related to a medical condition, the anxiety and avoidance must be clearly excessive.

Finally, to receive a diagnosis of agoraphobia, the clinician must determine that the symptoms are not better explained by another mental-health diagnosis. For example, if the person only avoids social situations, social anxiety disorder might be diagnosed. Other disorders associated with avoidance, such as major depression, specific phobias, and separation anxiety disorder, might be diagnosed instead of agoraphobia if symptoms are better accounted for by those disorders.

COURSE OF ILLNESS

Between one-third to one-half of people will have panic attacks prior to the onset of agoraphobia; the average age of onset for those individuals is late teens. For those who do not have panic attacks prior to the onset of agoraphobia, the average age of onset is later—in the mid to late 20's. While most develop the disorder at a younger age, a third of individuals will have an onset after age 40. Agoraphobia tends to be a chronic illness if left untreated. Most individuals with agoraphobia also have co-occurring psychiatric disorders, such as anxiety, mood, and/or substance-use disorders.

Agoraphobia

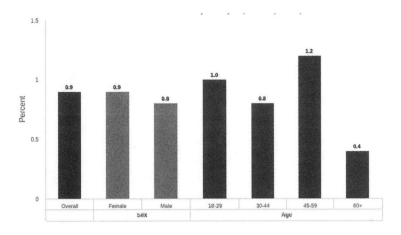

Figure 14.1. Past Year Prevalence of Agoraphobia among Adults (2001–2003)

PREVALENCE OF AGORAPHOBIA
Agoraphobia among Adults
- Based on diagnostic interview data from National Comorbidity Survey Replication (NCS-R), figure 14.1. shows past year prevalence of agoraphobia among U.S. adults 18 or older.
- An estimated 0.9 percent of U.S. adults had agoraphobia in the past year.
- Past year prevalence of agoraphobia among adults was similar for females (0.9%) and males (0.8%).
- An estimated 1.3 percent of U.S. adults experience agoraphobia at some time in their lives.

Agoraphobia with Impairment among Adult
- Of adults with agoraphobia in the past year degree of impairment ranged from mild-to-serious, as shown in figure 14.2. Impairment was determined by scores on the Sheehan Disability Scale.
- Of adults with agoraphobia in the past year, an estimated 40.6 percent had serious impairment, 30.7 percent had moderate impairment, and 28.7 percent had mild impairment.

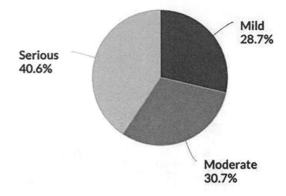

Figure 14.2. Past Year Severity of Agoraphobia with Impairment among Adult

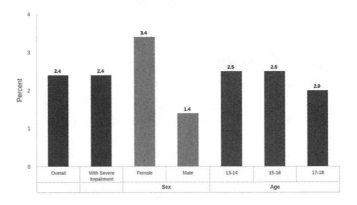

Figure 14.3. Lifetime Prevalence of Agoraphobia among Adolescents (2001–2004)

Lifetime Prevalence of Agoraphobia among Adolescents

- Based on diagnostic interview data from National Comorbidity Survey Adolescent Supplement (NCS-A), figure 14.3. shows lifetime prevalence of agoraphobia among U.S. adolescents 13 to 18 years of age.
- An estimated 2.4 percent of adolescents had agoraphobia at some time during their life, and all had severe impairment.
- The prevalence of agoraphobia among adolescents was higher for females (3.4%) than for males (1.4%).

Chapter 15 | Substance- or Medication-Induced Anxiety Disorder

Substance- or medication-induced anxiety disorder is diagnosed when a person experiences anxiety symptoms such as nervousness or panic attack by using or withdrawal from certain drugs, medication, or alcohol.

Whether it is speaking in front of a class or a job interview, we all feel a little anxious in our day to day lives. Public speaking often does not come naturally to many and it can be daunting to present a report in front of their classmates or give a speech. It may cause their breathing to become heavy and may give them sweaty palms. But after the task is over, they become normal again. Anxiety is our body's natural response to stress, and it comes and goes without interfering with our daily lives. But, if feelings of extreme nervousness or restlessness interrupt your daily activities and are prolonged over days and weeks, you might be having an anxiety disorder. Ironically, the medications or substances others use to calm their nerves may lead to medication-induced anxiety disorder in some people. Because most people think that substance use will help them feel good, they often do not consider that their substance use is elevating anxiety in them.

"Substance or Medication-Induced Anxiety Disorder," © 2020 Omnigraphics. Reviewed August 2020.

CAUSES OF SUBSTANCE- OR MEDICATION-INDUCED ANXIETY DISORDER

Our brain releases chemicals that help us to think, feel, and behave. An imbalance in these chemical levels alters our ability to act, feel, and think as we should. Alcohol and drugs like lysergic acid diethylamide (LSD) interfere with the brain's natural process of releasing chemicals and lead to substance-induced anxiety. In some cases, a person can experience anxiety for several weeks after they have stopped taking the drugs.

SYMPTOMS OF SUBSTANCE- OR MEDICATION-INDUCED ANXIETY DISORDER

The symptoms of substance- or medication-induced anxiety disorder occur while a person is currently on drugs (or alcohol) or has stopped using them. It includes:

- Difficulty in breathing
- Constantly thinking about how bad things are going to happen
- Constantly worrying that they will not get better
- Pain in the chest and pounding heartbeat
- Trouble with memory or concentration
- Cold sweats, tremors, chills
- Difficulty falling asleep at night
- Loss of appetite or stomach issues (diarrhea or vomiting)
- Fear losing grip on yourself and "losing it" (going crazy)

DRUGS AND SUBSTANCES THAT CAN CAUSE SUBSTANCE-INDUCED ANXIETY DISORDER

- Alcohol
- Marijuana
- Caffeine
- Sedatives
- Inhalants
- Opioids

- Cocaine
- Hallucinogens

FEW MEDICATIONS KNOWN TO CAUSE SUBSTANCE-INDUCED ANXIETY DISORDER

- Insulin
- Antidepressants
- Epinephrine
- Anesthetic
- Antipsychotics
- Corticosteroids
- Asthma medication
- Thyroid medication
- Seizure medication

HOW IS SUBSTANCE- OR MEDICATION-INDUCED ANXIETY DISORDER DIAGNOSED

Before making a diagnosis, the healthcare provider will make sure that you did not have anxiety before using substances and medications. Anxiety before substance abuse is not considered as substance-induced anxiety, even if that was what had made your symptoms worse. It is essential to be honest with the healthcare provider about the substances you have been using to make an effective treatment. The diagnosis process may include sharing your medical history, undergoing a physical exam, various tests and scans.

TREATMENT FOR SUBSTANCE- OR MEDICATION-INDUCED ANXIETY DISORDER

There is help available if you or someone you know is struggling with substance- or medication-induced anxiety disorder. With therapy and supervised detoxification, someone with a substance- or medication-induced anxiety disorder can overcome this condition. If any of your current medication is causing anxiety, reach out to your healthcare provider immediately. Do not be afraid to tell your healthcare provider if you have developed dependence over a particular medication or substance. Your healthcare provider will come up with a supervised detox treatment plan for you. The withdrawal period might seem complicated, but it is encouraged not to go back to using drugs or alcohol to deal with the withdrawal symptoms. The healthcare provider may choose to prescribe medication to help you cope during the withdrawal period. Stay the course and let them know if you face any difficulty following the treatment plan. Individual or group therapies are also helpful. A psychologist will help you identify any deep-seated issue you might be having that is causing you to be anxious. Being part of support groups such as Alcoholics Anonymous (AA) and Narcotics Anonymous (NA) also plays a huge role in the recovery process. Recovery may feel like a struggle, but sharing and listening to the stories of others who struggle with the same things you struggle with can help you realize you are not alone in this fight. Your healthcare provider can work alongside your counselor while coming up with your treatment plan.

References

1. "Substance-Induced Anxiety Disorder," Summit Medical Group, n.d.
2. Hartney, Elizabeth. "Substance/Medication-Induced Anxiety Disorder," Very Well Mind, February 2020.
3. Rosenker, Michelle. "What Is Substance-Induced Anxiety Disorder," Journey Pure Bowling Green, August 2019.
4. "Substance or Medication-Induced Anxiety Disorder," Pine Rest, n.d.
5. "What Meds Might Cause Anxiety," WebMD, n.d.
6. "Everything You Need to Know about Anxiety," Healthline, September 2018.

Part 3 | General Principles of Diagnosis and Treatment

Chapter 16 | **Ruling Out Medical Conditions with Anxiety as a Symptom**

According to the Anxiety and Depression Association of America (ADAA), 81.1 percent of the U.S. population 18 years of age and above, i.e., 40 million adults, are affected by anxiety disorders every year. Being anxious is part of our daily life, but when the feeling is prolonged and when it interferes with routine tasks, there might be an underlying cause for your anxiety. Sometimes various physical infirmities may mimic the symptoms of anxiety.

The following clues reveal if you have an underlying medical condition that is causing anxiety:

- You have never had anxiety disorder before and experience a sudden onset (anxiety disorders can be traced back to childhood).
- Your symptoms of anxiety vary.
- You do not have a history of anxiety disorders in your family.
- No significant changes (death of a loved one, moved to a new city or school, job change, etc. have taken place in your life.
- Symptoms of anxiety occur after sudden abnormalities in your vital signs.
- Anxiety symptoms occur alongside recent cognitive loss, headaches, visual disturbances, etc.
- You seem to be less alert and experience memory loss.

"Ruling Out Medical Conditions with Anxiety as a Symptom," © 2020 Omnigraphics. Reviewed August 2020.

- You have experienced anxiety symptoms while using certain medications and have changed medications.
- You are diagnosed with multiple medical conditions.

SOME OF THE REASONS FOR ANXIETY

When someone seeks help for anxiety disorders, they can have undiscovered medical conditions they are not yet tested for.

Tumors. Both brain and adrenal gland tumors can lead to various psychological symptoms such as anxiety, hallucinations, changes in personality, and physical symptoms, such as headaches and fatigue.

Hormonal imbalance. Thyroid malfunction, such as overactive thyroid (hyperthyroidism) or underactive thyroid (hypothyroidism) can also cause anxiety symptoms similar to a panic attack—increased heart rate that causes you to breathe fast and sweat more, raising body temperature. Estrogen in females also acts as a trigger for anxiety, especially during menopause, or if the cycle fluctuates.

Infectious diseases. These can sometimes trigger anxiety as a result of the disease. For instance, a person can develop a neurological tic seen with an anxiety disorder due to strep infection that has been left untreated. Lyme disease in the second stage can also trigger neurological and psychological symptoms.

Nutrition. One of the most common causes of anxiety is anemia (iron deficiency). Because your body is not receiving enough oxygen from the red blood cells (RBCs), your pulse increases to make up for the oxygen loss causing you to feel anxious. Lack of Vitamin B_{12} can also mimic anxiety symptoms.

Central nervous system (CNS). Anxiety symptoms such as dizziness, disorientation, and headache can occur due to severe head trauma, or a mild concussion, vertigo, or even migraine. Chronic illnesses, such as Alzheimer disease (AD) and Guillain-Barré syndrome can also lead to anxiety disorders.

Electrolyte abnormalities and environmental toxins. Certain medications may alter your electrolyte and cause anxiety. Prolonged exposure to insecticides (organophosphates) may also cause anxiety symptoms.

Drugs. Many over-the-counter (OTC) medicines, prescription drugs, homeopathic medicine, and illicit drugs can cause anxiety symptoms. Contact your healthcare provider if you experience symptoms of anxiety after using the prescribed medications. If you are going through an alcohol or drug withdrawal period, you might experience symptoms of anxiety.

Diabetes. According to the Centers for Disease Control and Prevention (CDC), people with diabetes are 20 percent more likey to experience anxiety than people who do not have diabetes. Rise and fall in blood sugar levels can lead to symptoms similar to an anxiety attack such as dizziness, sweating, and breathlessness.

Asthma. Those diagnosed with asthma may be at risk for developing anxiety due to asthma attacks. Someone who never had asthma might confuse shortness of breath with anxiety rather than adult-onset asthma.

Sleep apnea. Similar to anxiety symptoms, if you wake up breathless or with your heart racing, you might have a condition called "sleep apnea."

Lack of sleep. Chronic insomnia and sleep deprivation can increase individuals' chances to acquire anxiety-related disorders.

Fibromyalgia. Often addressed as "invisible illness," symptoms of fibromyalgia mimic that of anxiety disorder or arthritis as its classic symptoms are fatigue and pain in joints and muscles. Other symptoms are feelings of worry, mood swings, insomnia, or twitching, to name a few. Doctors do not know what causes fibromyalgia, and there is no test to diagnose it, and so it is often misdiagnosed as anxiety.

Polycystic ovary syndrome (PCOS). Women suffering from PCOS can feel anxious, irritable, fatigued, and experience changes in mood due to hormonal imbalance.

Endometriosis. A painful disorder where the lining found inside the uterus grows outside the uterus and is often misdiagnosed as anxiety when women experience pelvic pain. This condition is still not widely known among doctors and leads to misdiagnosis.

Postural orthostatic tachycardia syndrome (POTS). Characterized by but not limited to a rapid heart rate, drop in blood pressure, chest pain, and shortness of breath, POTS is a type of an autonomic nervous system disorder that can be misdiagnosed as anxiety.

Inappropriate sinus tachycardia (IST). Sometimes mistaken for POTS, although both disorders are distinct, IST causes the heart to beat rapidly and can be misdiagnosed as anxiety.

Adrenal insufficiency. Adrenal glands produce a hormone called "cortisol." Low cortisol levels can cause depression and anxiety, although more evaluation is required to see if a hormonal imbalance or mental illness causes these.

Crohn disease. Symptoms for Crohn disease can be mistaken for anxiety as anxiety can cause gastrointestinal problems similar to Crohn disease (constipation, diarrheal, stomach ache, etc.). Crohn disease is an inflammatory bowel syndrome caused by bacteria or viruses that triggers the body's autoimmune response or caused by genes.

Miscellaneous. Chronic and rare diseases such as Wilson disease, lupus, rheumatoid arthritis (RA), Huntington disease, and seizure disorder can also present anxiety and other psychological symptoms.

References

1. "Facts and Statistic," Anxiety and Depression Association of America (ADAA), n.d.
2. Cain, Robert. "Is a Hidden Medical Condition Causing Your Anxiety?" Cleveland Clinic, June 2018.
3. Feintuch, Stacey. "12 Medical Conditions That Could Cause or Trigger Anxiety," February 2020.
4. Easton-Smith, Kim. "10 Physical Conditions That Could Be Causing Your Anxiety," April 2018.
5. Migdol, Erin. "10 Conditions That May Be Misdiagnosed as Anxiety," The Mighty, July 2018.

Chapter 17 | **Diagnostic Tools for Anxiety Disorders**

Anxiety is a common and natural emotion caused by the brain when reacting to stress or any potential threat or danger. People usually worry and feel anxious about health, financial situations, taking a test, facing a problem, or even before making important decisions. Occasional anxiety is normal, but when a person is constantly worried, afraid, or overwhelmed over minor situations, it may be due to a form of mental illness. Such a mental condition is referred to as "anxiety disorder." Excessive anxiety disorder can make a person avoid social gatherings, work, school, and even family get-togethers.

DIAGNOSIS OF ANXIETY DISORDER

The diagnosis for anxiety is not simple, as complete physical examination is essential so that the doctor can discover or rule out any illness that may cause symptoms of anxiety. Personal history or family history is also an important, and for the same reason, it is best to be honest with the doctor. Certain reasons, such as the below, can cause generalized anxiety disorder (GAD):

- Alcohol consumption
- Medications
- Hormonal imbalance
- Physical, mental, or verbal abuse

"Diagnostic Tools for Anxiety Disorders," © 2020 Omnigraphics. Reviewed August 2020.

GAD-7

The GAD-7 is a tool used to assess the severity of GAD in a person. This seven-point diagnostic tool allows an individual to rate the severity of GAD in the person over the weeks. It takes only a couple of minutes to answer the questionnaire, which is then calculated with assigned scores for each answer. The total score for the seven questions ranges from 0–21.

- People scoring below 10 are diagnosed with mild anxiety
- People scoring 10–15 are diagnosed with moderate anxiety
- People scoring above 15 are diagnosed with severe anxiety

Further evaluation is required if a person scores above 10 points.

BECK ANXIETY INVENTORY

The Beck Anxiety Inventory (BAI) is a tool that explains 21 signs of anxiety, such as "wobbling in the legs," "scared," and "fear of losing control." Patients are asked to assess how much any of these symptoms have affected them over the last week, on a scale ranging from 0 (not at all) to 63 (seriously). The overall score is at least 0 and at most 63. Patients who scored a higher number were said to have an increased level of anxiety disorder. The scores may range from 0 to 63.

- Minimal anxiety levels (0–7)
- Mild anxiety (8–15)
- Moderate anxiety (16–25)
- Severe anxiety (26–63)

The method has been confirmed in a study of 160 clinical out-patients with various anxiety and depressive conditions.

THE STATE-TRAIT ANXIETY INVENTORY

The State-Trait Anxiety Inventory (STAI) tool developed by Spielberger et al. is used to identify and measure the presence and severity of anxiety symptoms. It is available in two different versions, which are used for adults and children. The tool has two subscales:

The State Anxiety Scale (S-anxiety) assesses the present state of anxiety by understanding how respondents feel at the moment using elements that measure individual sensations of discomfort, stress, nervousness, concern by activating the nervous system. The S-Anxiety scale answers the intensity of current feelings with options such as:

1. Not at all
2. Maybe
3. Somewhat so
4. Very much so

The Trait Anxiety Scale (T-Anxiety) measures fairly stable aspects of "proneness of anxiety," including the general state of composure, trust, and comfort. T-Anxiety scale responses measure the level of emotions, such as:

1. Almost rarely
2. At times
3. Sometimes
4. Almost always

ANXIETY SENSITIVITY

Anxiety Sensitivity is associated with heart attacks, insomnia, and other common psychiatric illnesses. It is usually viewed as a relatively stable characteristic. The Anxiety Sensitivity Index (ASI) is a scale of 16 items that includes elements which identify specific worries someone may have about their anxiety. The Anxiety Sensitivity Index-3 for Anxiety (ASI-3) is a scale of 18 items.

Each item is rated by selecting one of five phrases:

- 0 points—very little
- 1 point—a little
- 2 points—a few or some
- 3 points—many or much
- 4 points—too many or very much

SOCIAL ANXIETY QUESTIONNAIRE

The Social Anxiety Questionnaire (SAQ) is a new measure of social anxiety for adults. The structure of the questionnaire was supported by a 5-factor analysis and was labeled as:

1. Encounters with strangers
2. Public speech/conversation with influential individuals
3. Encounters with the same sex
4. Disapproval and humiliation
5. Assertive display of irritation, resentment, or dissatisfaction

PENN STATE WORRY QUESTIONNAIRE

The Penn State Worry Questionnaire (PSWQ) is a self-report questionnaire consisting of 16 items. It measures the intensity and frequency of chronic and uncontrollable worry. The PSWQ comprises questions that inquire about various facets of anxiety, and each item is measured on a 5-point Likert scale (a psychometric scale used to measure responses to a statement).

KOREAN ANXIETY SCREENING ASSESSMENT

The Korean Anxiety Screening Assessment K-ANX is a newly formed test to screen anxiety disorders by researchers. A GAD object bank consisting of 273 items is constructed to develop the K-ANX. From this, eleven items were selected considering various criteria.

References

1. "Generalized Anxiety Disorder: When Worry Gets Out of Control," National Institute of Mental Health, January 21, 2011.
2. "Is the Beck Anxiety Inventory a Good Tool to Assess the Severity of Anxiety?" National Center for Biotechnology Information, July 4, 2011.
3. Julian, Laura J. "Measures of Anxiety," National Center for Biotechnology Information, November 9, 2011.

4. Hovenkamp H.M, Johanna. "Anxiety Sensitivity, Its Stability and Longitudinal Association with Severity of Anxiety Symptoms," Springer Nature, March 13, 2019.
5. "Psychometric Properties of an Innovative Self-Report Measure: The Social Anxiety Questionnaire for Adults," National Center for Biotechnology Information (NCBI), March 16, 2015.
6. Kim, Yeseul; Park, Yeonsoo. "Psychometric Properties of an Innovative Self-Report Measure: The Social Anxiety Questionnaire for Adults," National Center for Biotechnology Information (NCBI), November 22, 2018.
7. "Generalised Anxiety Disorder Assessment (GAD-7)," Child Outcomes Research Consortium, June 2020.
8. Robert L. "Spitzer et al.," *Archives of Internal Medicine*, 2006.

Chapter 18 | Introduction to Treatment Options for People with Anxiety

Anxiety disorders are generally treated with psychotherapy, medication, or both. There are many ways to treat anxiety and people should work with their doctor to choose the treatment that is best for them.

PSYCHOTHERAPY
Psychotherapy or "talk therapy" can help people with anxiety disorders. To be effective, psychotherapy must be directed at the person's specific anxieties and tailored to her or his needs.

Cognitive-Behavioral Therapy
Cognitive-behavioral therapy (CBT) is an example of one type of psychotherapy that can help people with anxiety disorders. It teaches people different ways of thinking, behaving, and reacting to anxiety-producing and fearful objects and situations. CBT can also help people learn and practice social skills, which is vital for treating social anxiety disorder.

Cognitive therapy and exposure therapy are two CBT methods that are often used, together or by themselves, to treat social anxiety disorder. Cognitive therapy focuses on identifying, challenging, and then neutralizing unhelpful or distorted thoughts underlying anxiety disorders. Exposure therapy focuses on confronting

This chapter includes text excerpted from "Anxiety Disorders," National Institute of Mental Health (NIMH), July 2018.

the fears underlying an anxiety disorder to help people engage in activities they have been avoiding. Exposure therapy is sometimes used along with relaxation exercises and/or imagery.

Cognitive-behavioral therapy can be conducted individually or with a group of people who have similar difficulties. Often "homework" is assigned for participants to complete between sessions.

MEDICATION

Medication does not cure anxiety disorders but can help relieve symptoms. Medication for anxiety is prescribed by doctors, such as a psychiatrist or primary care provider. Some states also allow psychologists who have received specialized training to prescribe psychiatric medications. The most common classes of medications used to combat anxiety disorders are antianxiety drugs (such as benzodiazepines), antidepressants, and beta-blockers.

Antianxiety Medications

Antianxiety medications can help reduce the symptoms of anxiety, panic attacks, or extreme fear and worry. The most common antianxiety medications are called "benzodiazepines." Although benzodiazepines are sometimes used as first-line treatments for generalized anxiety disorder (GAD), they have both benefits and drawbacks.

Some benefits of benzodiazepines are that they are effective in relieving anxiety and take effect more quickly than antidepressant medications often prescribed for anxiety. Some drawbacks of benzodiazepines are that people can build up a tolerance to them if they are taken over a long period of time and they may need higher and higher doses to get the same effect. Some people may even become dependent on them.

To avoid these problems, doctors usually prescribe benzodiazepines for short periods of time, a practice that is especially helpful for older adults, people who have substance-abuse problems, and people who become dependent on medication easily.

If people suddenly stop taking benzodiazepines, they may have withdrawal symptoms, or their anxiety may return. Therefore, benzodiazepines should be tapered off slowly. When you and your doctor have decided it is time to stop the medication, the doctor will help you slowly and safely decrease your dose.

For long-term use, benzodiazepines are often considered a second-line treatment for anxiety (with antidepressants being considered a first-line treatment) as well as an "as-needed" treatment for any distressing flare-ups of symptoms.

A different type of antianxiety medication is buspirone. It is a nonbenzodiazepine medication specifically indicated for the treatment of chronic anxiety, although it does not help everyone.

Antidepressants

Antidepressants are used to treat depression, but they can also be helpful for treating anxiety disorders. They may help improve the way your brain uses certain chemicals that control mood or stress. You may need to try several different antidepressant medicines before finding the one that improves your symptoms and has manageable side effects. A medication that has helped you or a close family member in the past will often be considered.

Antidepressants can take time to work, so it is important to give the medication a chance before reaching a conclusion about its effectiveness. If you begin taking antidepressants, do not stop taking them without the help of a doctor. When you and your doctor have decided it is time to stop the medication, the doctor will help you slowly and safely decrease your dose. Stopping them abruptly can cause withdrawal symptoms.

Antidepressants called "selective serotonin reuptake inhibitors" (SSRIs) and "serotonin-norepinephrine reuptake inhibitors" (SNRIs) are commonly used as first-line treatments for anxiety. Less-commonly used—but effective—treatments for anxiety disorders are older classes of antidepressants, such as tricyclic antidepressants and monoamine oxidase inhibitors (MAOIs).

Beta-Blockers

Although beta-blockers are most often used to treat high blood pressure, they can also be used to help relieve the physical symptoms of anxiety, such as rapid heartbeat, shaking, trembling, and blushing. These medications, when taken for a short period of time, can help people keep physical symptoms under control. They can also be used "as-needed" to reduce acute anxiety, including as a preventive intervention for some predictable forms of performance anxieties.

Choosing the Right Medication

Some types of drugs may work better for specific types of anxiety disorders, so people should work closely with their doctor to identify which medication is best for them. Certain substances such as caffeine, some over-the-counter (OTC) cold medicines, illicit drugs, and herbal supplements may aggravate the symptoms of anxiety disorders or interact with prescribed medication. Patients should talk with their doctor, so they can learn which substances are safe and which to avoid.

Choosing the right medication, medication dose, and treatment plan should be done under an expert's care and should be based on a person's needs and their medical situation. Your doctor may try several medicines before finding the right one.

You and your doctor should discuss:

- How well medications are working or might work to improve your symptoms
- Benefits and side effects of each medication
- Risk for serious side effects based on your medical history
- The likelihood of the medications requiring lifestyle changes
- Costs of each medication
- Other alternative therapies, medications, vitamins, and supplements you are taking and how these may affect your treatment; a combination of medication and psychotherapy is the best approach for many people with anxiety disorders
- How the medication should be stopped (Some drugs cannot be stopped abruptly and must be tapered off slowly under a doctor's supervision).

SUPPORT GROUPS

Some people with anxiety disorders might benefit from joining a self-help or support group and sharing their problems and achievements with others. Internet chat rooms might also be useful, but any advice received over the Internet should be used with caution, as Internet acquaintances have usually never seen each other and what has helped one person is not necessarily what is best for another. You should always check with your doctor before following any treatment advice found on the Internet. Talking with a trusted friend or member of the clergy can also provide support, but it is not necessarily a sufficient alternative to care from a doctor or other health professional.

STRESS MANAGEMENT TECHNIQUES

Stress management techniques and meditation can help people with anxiety disorders calm themselves and may enhance the effects of therapy. Research suggests that aerobic exercise can help some people manage their anxiety; however, exercise should not take the place of standard care and more research is needed.

Chapter 19 | **Psychotherapy**

Psychotherapy (sometimes called "talk therapy") is a term for a variety of treatment techniques that aim to help a person identify and change troubling emotions, thoughts, and behavior. Most psychotherapy takes place with a licensed and trained mental-healthcare professional and a patient meeting one-on-one or with other patients in a group setting.

Someone might seek out psychotherapy for different reasons:

- You might be dealing with severe or long-term stress from a job or family situation, the loss of a loved one, or relationship or other family issues. Or you may have symptoms with no physical explanation: changes in sleep or appetite, low energy, a lack of interest or pleasure in activities that you once enjoyed, persistent irritability, or a sense of discouragement or hopelessness that will not go away.
- A health professional may suspect or have diagnosed a condition such as depression, bipolar disorder, posttraumatic stress or other disorder and recommended psychotherapy as a first treatment or to go along with medication.
- You may be seeking treatment for a family member or child who has been diagnosed with a condition affecting mental health and for whom a health professional has recommended treatment.

An exam by your primary care practitioner can ensure there is nothing in your overall health that would explain your or a loved one's symptoms.

This chapter includes text excerpted from "Psychotherapies," National Institute of Mental Health (NIMH), November 2016. Reviewed August 2020.

WHAT TO CONSIDER WHEN LOOKING FOR A THERAPIST

Therapists have different professional backgrounds and specialties.

There are many different types of psychotherapy. Different therapies are often variations on an established approach, such as cognitive-behavioral therapy (CBT). There is no formal approval process for psychotherapies as there is for the use of medications in medicine. For many therapies, however, research involving large numbers of patients has provided evidence that treatment is effective for specific disorders. These "evidence-based therapies" (EBTs) have been shown in research to reduce symptoms of depression, anxiety, and other disorders.

The particular approach a therapist uses depends on the condition being treated and the training and experience of the therapist. Also, therapists may combine and adapt elements of different approaches.

One goal of establishing an evidence base for psychotherapies is to prevent situations in which a person receives therapy for months or years with no benefit. If you have been in therapy and feel you are not getting better, talk to your therapist, or look into other practitioners or approaches. The object of therapy is to gain relief from symptoms and improve quality of life (QOL).

Once you have identified one or more possible therapists, a preliminary conversation with a therapist can help you get an idea of how treatment will proceed and whether you feel comfortable with the therapist. Rapport and trust are important. Discussions in therapy are deeply personal and it is important that you feel comfortable with the therapist and have trust and confidence in her or his expertise. Consider asking the following questions:

- What are the credentials and experience of the therapist? Does she or he have a specialty?
- What approach will the therapist take to help you? Does she or he practice a particular type of therapy? What can the therapist tell you about the rationale for the therapy and the evidence base?
- Does the therapist have experience in diagnosing and treating the age group (e.g., a child) and the specific condition for which treatment is being sought? If a

child is the patient, how will parents be involved in treatment?

- What are the goals of therapy? Does the therapist recommend a specific time frame or number of sessions? How will progress be assessed and what happens if you (or the therapist) feel you are not starting to feel better?
- Will there be homework?
- Are medications an option? How will medications be prescribed if the therapist is not an M.D.?
- Are your meetings confidential? How can this be assured?

Psychotherapies and Other Treatment Options

Psychotherapy can be an alternative to medication or can be used along with other treatment options, such as medications. Choosing the right treatment plan should be based on a person's individual needs and medical situation and under a mental-health professional's care.

Even when medications relieve symptoms, psychotherapy and other interventions can help a person address specific issues. These might include self-defeating ways of thinking, fears, problems with interactions with other people, or dealing with situations at home and at school or with employment.

Elements of Psychotherapy

A variety of different kinds of psychotherapies and interventions have been shown to be effective for specific disorders. Psychotherapists may use one primary approach, or incorporate different elements depending on their training, the condition being treated, and the needs of the person receiving treatment.

Here are examples of the elements that psychotherapies can include:
- Helping a person become aware of ways of thinking that may be automatic but are inaccurate and harmful. (An example might be someone who has a low

opinion of her or his own abilities.) The therapist helps the person find ways to question these thoughts, understand how they affect emotions and behavior, and try ways to change self-defeating patterns. This approach is central to cognitive-behavioral therapy.

- Identifying ways to cope with stress
- Examining in-depth a person's interactions with others and offering guidance with social and communication skills, if needed
- Relaxation and mindfulness techniques
- Exposure therapy for people with anxiety disorders. In exposure therapy, a person spends brief periods, in a supportive environment, learning to tolerate the distress certain items, ideas, or imagined scenes cause. Over time the fear associated with these things dissipates.
- Tracking emotions and activities and the impact of each on the other
- Safety planning can include helping a person recognize warning signs, and thinking about coping strategies such as contacting friends, family, or emergency personnel
- Supportive counseling to help a person explore troubling issues and provide emotional support

eHealth

The telephone, Internet, and mobile devices have opened up new possibilities for providing interventions that can reach people in areas where mental-health professionals may not be easily available, and can be at hand 24/7. Some of these approaches involve a therapist providing help at a distance, but others—such as web-based programs and cell phone apps—are designed to provide information and feedback in the absence of a therapist.

Some approaches that use electronic media to provide help for mental-health-related conditions have been shown by research to be helpful in some situations, others not as yet. The American Psychological Association (APA) has information to consider before choosing online therapy.

If you are interested in using a mobile app, read the accompanying information, including whether and how the app has been tested. If you are working with a therapist, consult with her or him for help in evaluating the app.

TAKING THE FIRST STEP

The symptoms of mental disorders can have a profound effect on someone's QOL and ability to function. Treatment can address symptoms as well as assist someone experiencing severe or ongoing stress. Some of the reasons that you might consider seeking out psychotherapy include:

- Overwhelming sadness or helplessness that does not go away
- Serious, unusual insomnia or sleeping too much
- Difficulty focusing on work, or carrying out other everyday activities
- Constant worry and anxiety
- Drinking to excess or any behavior that harms self or others
- Dealing with a difficult transition such as a divorce, children leaving home, job difficulties, or the death of someone close
- Children's behavior problems that interfere with school, family, or peers

Seeking help is not an admission of weakness, but a step towards understanding and obtaining relief from distressing symptoms.

FINDING A THERAPIST

Many different professionals offer psychotherapy. Examples include psychiatrists, psychologists, social workers, counselors, and psychiatric nurses. Information on the credentials of providers is available from the National Alliance on Mental Illness (NAMI).

Your health plan may have a list of mental-health practitioners who participate in the plan. Other resources on the "Help for Mental Illnesses" page can help you look for reduced-cost health services. The resources listed there include links to help find reduced-cost treatment. When talking with a prospective therapist, ask about treatment fees, whether the therapist participates in insurance plans, and whether there is a sliding scale for fees according to income.

University or medical school-affiliated programs may offer treatment options. Search on the website of local university health centers for their psychiatry or psychology departments.

You can also go to the website of your state or county government and search for the health department for information on mental-health related programs within your state.

Chapter 20 | **Cognitive-Behavioral Therapy**

WHAT IS COGNITIVE-BEHAVIORAL THERAPY?

Cognitive-behavioral therapy (CBT) is a structured, time-limited, present-focused approach to psychotherapy that helps patients develop strategies to modify dysfunctional thinking patterns or cognitions (i.e., the "C" in CBT) and maladaptive emotions and behaviors (i.e., the "B" in CBT) in order to assist them in resolving current problems. A typical course of CBT is approximately 16 sessions, in which patients are seen on a weekly or biweekly basis. CBT was originally developed to treat depression, and it has since been adapted to the treatment of anxiety disorders, substance-use disorders, personality disorders, eating disorders, bipolar disorder, and even schizophrenia. Many patients show substantial improvement after 4 to 18 sessions of CBT. Contemporary research shows that CBT is efficacious in treating mild, moderate, and severe mental-health symptoms, that it is equally as efficacious as psychotropic medications in the short-term, and that it is more efficacious than psychotropic medications in the long-term. There is a great deal of research supporting CBT's efficacy for treating an array of mental disorders using both individual and group formats.

GENERAL SESSION STRUCTURE

Cognitive-behavioral therapy follows a session structure in order to make efficient use of time, ensure that goals are achieved in each

This chapter includes text excerpted from "Cognitive Behavioral Therapy for Depression in Veterans and Military Servicemembers," Mental Illness Research, Education and Clinical Centers (MIRECC), U.S. Department of Veterans Affairs (VA), April 30, 2011. Reviewed August 2020; Text under the heading "Exposure Therapy" is © 2020 Omnigraphics. Reviewed August 2020.

session, and maintain a thread across sessions so that progress is made toward long-term goals. The components of CBT session structure include:

- A brief mood check
- A bridge from the previous session
- The setting of an agenda
- A review of the previous session's homework assignment
- A discussion of agenda items
- Periodic summaries
- A homework assignment
- A final summary and feedback

This structure models for patients is an adaptive problem-solving approach and communicates hope that their problems can be addressed in a systematic manner. Of course, sound clinical judgment might point to an alternative course of action during a session that should be pursued in specific situations, such as in response to crises or when patients report or display behaviors that suggest a specific action should be taken to assess or address potential suicide risk.

Cognitive-behavioral therapists are strongly encouraged to be cognizant of the therapeutic relationship as they structure the session. CBT is fundamentally a collaborative enterprise between the therapist and the patient. Patients are active participants in all aspects of therapy and contribute to the structure of therapy as much as is possible (e.g., helping to set the agenda, developing homework assignments). It is found that many patients welcome the CBT session structure so that expectations for what will be accomplished and their roles in treatment are clear. However, some patients have an adverse reaction to the session structure. Jack, for example, believed that therapy is a time to "vent frustrations" and found it offensive that his therapist wanted to "take care of business" before letting him "get things off of his chest." For this reason, early socialization to CBT and discussion of the therapy process are important. Furthermore, in some instances, such as that with Jack, therapists are encouraged to be creative in modifying session structure to respond to the preferences of patients in order to foster a strong, collaborative therapeutic relationship, which should always take precedence. In Jack's case, he and his therapist agreed that he could spend the first 10 to 15 minutes of each session "venting" about the previous week, and then they would move onto the other CBT session components.

Brief Mood Check

At the beginning of each session, the therapist briefly assesses patients' mood in the time since the previous session. The purpose of the brief mood check is to track patients' progress over time and to make this progress explicit so that it instills hope and builds momentum. It also alerts the therapist to symptoms that require immediate attention in session (e.g., a patient who endorses suicide ideation accompanied by a plan in the time since the previous session). One way to facilitate the brief mood check is to have patients arrive 5 to 10 minutes before their sessions and complete a standardized self-report inventory. The therapist can scan patients' responses to such an inventory and ask follow-up questions about symptoms that show improvement or decline, or about symptoms that have been the most concerning for patients in the past.

The most commonly used self-report inventory for this purpose is the Beck Depression Inventory-II. It is a 21-item self-report instrument developed to measure the severity of depression in adults and older adults in the previous one or two weeks. The measure assumes that the respondent is able to read at an 8th-grade reading level; for patients who cannot read at this level, therapists can administer the measure orally. Each item consists of four statements reflecting increasing levels of severity of a particular symptom of depression. The score for each individual item ranges from 0 to 3. The total score ranges from 0 to 63 and is achieved by adding the 21 ratings. If more than one statement for an item is endorsed, then the statement with the highest score is selected for that item. The BDI manual provides interpretation guidelines on the severity of depression based on total BDI score: 0–13 (minimal), 14–19 (mild), 20–28 (moderate), and 29–63 (severe). These scoring guidelines were established for adult patients who were seeking outpatient mental-health services; therefore, therapists are cautioned to interpret these scores with respect to the clinical sample and setting in which the measure is used.

Although, in general, higher total BDI scores are associated with increased risk of suicide, special attention should be paid to two particular items. If the patient endorses a 1 or higher on the suicide item (Item 9) or a 2 or higher on the hopelessness item (Item 2), then further assessment of suicide risk may be warranted. Thus, the completion and evaluation of the BDI at each therapy session provides the therapist with one strategy for monitoring ongoing suicide risk.

FINAL SUMMARY AND FEEDBACK

At the end of session, the therapist conducts a final summary or, alternatively, has the patient summarize the most important lessons gleaned from the session. In obtaining feedback about the session, questions such as if the session was helpful should be avoided by the therapist. It has been observed that, patients will usually respond that the session was helpful. Although such responses may be reassuring to the therapist, they do not necessarily facilitate the treatment. Rather, it is suggested that the therapist asks questions such as "What was the most helpful thing that we discussed in today's session?" or "What will you take away from this session?" Asking for feedback in this manner allows for the therapist to gain a better understanding of the specific points that resonated most with the patient. Therapists should also ask about how the patient felt about the session, especially if a particularly upsetting or sensitive topic was discussed. This is an important question to ask because patients may avoid future sessions if they leave sessions feeling distressed and do not have a plan for dealing with this distress. The therapist can also assess whether the patient thinks she or he was understood correctly and whether she or he wants to do anything differently in the next session. Items not discussed in this session could be identified at this point and established as agenda items for the following week. The therapist writes down this feedback and is sure to introduce the items identified by the patient in the next session.

INITIAL PHASE OF TREATMENT

The initial phase of treatment can last as few as one session and as many as three sessions. The main goals of the initial phase of treatment are to:

- Conduct an initial clinical assessment
- Motivate patients for change
- Socialize patients into treatment, including helping them to understand the structure and process of CBT
- Establish clear treatment goals

During the initial sessions, the therapist works to form a sound working alliance with patients that will serve as a basis to develop a case conceptualization and to implement the behavioral and cognitive interventions. In other words, during the initial sessions, the therapist makes interventions that will set the stage for success in the middle phase of treatment. The patient, in turn, assents to treatment, communicating a commitment to working on her or his problems within the CBT framework.

MIDDLE PHASE OF TREATMENT

During the middle phase of treatment, the patient and therapist work together to address the treatment goals established in the initial sessions in a systematic, strategic manner. The therapist uses a combination of cognitive and behavioral strategies as indicated by the case conceptualization. However, the therapist also continues to remain cognizant about the strength of the therapeutic relationship and balances relationship-building strategies with cognitive- and behavioral-change strategies, as necessary. Many Veterans achieve the greatest amount of success when they first make tangible behavioral changes in their lives, which puts them in a better place to examine and evaluate their thoughts and beliefs using cognitive strategies. Although these strategies primarily occur in the middle phase of treatment, therapists are encouraged to use them when relevant in the initial phase of treatment so that patients notice symptom change as immediately as possible.

LATER PHASE OF THIS TREATMENT

The main focus during the later phase of this treatment is to evaluate patients' progress toward their treatment goals and whether they have learned and can apply specific skills that may help to reduce or prevent a relapse of depression. Usually, the later phase of treatment occurs following an adequate dose of treatment (usually 12 to 16 sessions). However, given the flexible nature of this protocol, the later phase of treatment may occur after patients have attended a fewer number of sessions, or it may occur after the patient has attended more than 16 sessions. In this part of the manual, the Mental Illness Research, Education and Clinical Centers (MIRECC) presents some guidelines for assisting therapists in determining whether patients are clinically ready for the later phase of treatment. As with other aspects of CBT, it is recommended that the termination or tapering of CBT sessions is collaboratively decided between the therapist and patient. There are three main tasks that the therapist undertakes in the later phase of CBT for depressed patients:

- Reviewing progress toward treatment goals
- Summarizing and consolidating skills learned during the middle phase of treatment, including preventing future lapses of depression
- Additional treatment planning

EXPOSURE THERAPY

The exposure therapy is one of the most effective treatments for anxiety disorders. Through this treatment plan, the psychologist helps to refrain a person's brain from sending fear signals when there is no danger. It requires the person to confront their fear(s) and to overcome anxiety rather than just avoiding situations or places that make them anxious. Avoiding stressful situations or things that make a person afraid might seem to prevent one from experiencing an anxiety attack, but in the long term can make the anxiety disorder worse. The psychologist creates a safe space where the patient is "exposed" to what they fear to break the chain of avoidance and fear. When the patient is exposed to their fear in a safe environment, it reduces fear in them. Range of anxiety disorders that can be treated by exposure therapy are as follows:

- Panic disorder (PD)
- Phobias
- Generalized anxiety disorder (GAD)
- Social anxiety disorder (SAD)
- Posttraumatic stress disorder (PTSD)
- Obsessive-compulsive disorder (OCD)

Variations of Exposure Therapy

The idea behind exposure therapy is to repeatedly expose the patients to their fears or situations to gain control of the situation and diminish their anxiety. This can be done in two ways. The first one is called "in vivo exposure," where the psychologist makes the patient directly face their fears or put them in situations that make them anxious. For instance, someone who is afraid of spiders may be asked to hold one under supervision. The other approach is called "imaginal exposure," where the psychologist may ask the person to imagine a situation that scares them rather than making them face it in real life.

Another way to help patients overcome their anxiety is through virtual reality (VR) technology—with a simulated experience that can be similar to or completely different from the real world—where in vivo experience is not practical. For example, if someone is afraid of heights and is not ready to climb up the stairs of a high-rise building, they can still experience and be exposed to climbing up the stairs by merely putting on a VR headset. Another variation of exposure therapy is "interoceptive exposure." Some individuals fear harmless sensations like a rapid heartbeat. To help them overcome this fear, the psychologist may make the person run to speed up their heart rate, teaching that it is harmless.

References

1. "What Is Exposure Therapy," American Psychology Association (APA), July 2017.
2. Carbonell, Dave. "Exposure Therapy for Fears and Phobias," The Anxiety Coach, July 2020.
3. Smith, Melinda; Segal, Robert; Segal, Jeanne. "Therapy for Anxiety Disorders," Help Guide, November 2019.

Chapter 21 | **Antianxiety and Sedative Medications**

Antianxiety and sedative medications are drugs primarily used to reduce anxiety and chronic overarousal, and to facilitate sleep. These medications are widely prescribed, both to persons with a psychiatric disorder and to those in distress but without a specific psychiatric disorder. Antianxiety and sedative drugs are used with a variety of different psychiatric disorders, usually in combination with other medications.

DIFFERENT TYPES OF MEDICATIONS

Antianxiety and sedative medications can be divided into two broad classes of drugs: Antianxiety medications and sedative-hypnotics (the term "hypnotic" refers to sleep-inducing). All of these drugs have clinical effects on both reducing anxiety and causing sedation, although antianxiety drugs have the most specific effect on anxiety. Unlike many other medications for psychiatric disorders, the effects of these drugs are quite rapid and require only one to two hours to take effect. These different types of medication are described below.

Antianxiety Medications

The most common type of antianxiety drugs is the chemical class of benzodiazepines. In addition to relieving severe symptoms of anxiety, these drugs also relax the muscles and cause mild sedation.

This chapter includes text excerpted from "Facts about Antianxiety and Sedative Medications," Mental Illness Research, Education and Clinical Centers (MIRECC), U.S. Department of Veterans Affairs (VA), May 25, 2013. Reviewed August 2020.

Table 21.1. List of Antianxiety Medications

Long-Acting Benzodiazepines (More than 24-Hour Half-Life)		
Brand Name	**Chemical**	**Average Daily Dosage (mg/day)**
Valium	diazepam	2–60
Librium	chlordiazepoxide	15–100
Centrax	prazepam	20–60
Klonopin	clonazepam	0.5–20
Short Acting Benzodiazepines (Less than 24-Hour Half-Life)		
Brand Name	**Chemical**	**Average Daily Dosage (mg/day)**
Serax	oxazepam	30–120
Ativan	lorazepam	0.5–10
Xanax	alprazolam	0.5–6
Other Antianxiety Medications		
Brand Name	**Chemical**	**Average Daily Dosage (mg/day)**
Buspar	buspirone	2–60

Many different types of benzodiazepines exist. Another common antianxiety medication is Buspar (buspirone), which is a different chemical class from the benzodiazepines. Antidepressant medications are sometimes also used for the treatment of anxiety, such as obsessive-compulsive disorder (OCD).

The clinical effects of the different types of benzodiazepines on anxiety are the same. However, the drugs differ in how long they remain in the body (measured by how long it takes for the body to excrete half of the drug, i.e., the drug's half-life). Some benzodiazepines remain in the body for relatively brief periods of time (such as Xanax, with a half-life of twelve hours), while others remain much longer (such as Valium, with a half-life of sixty hours). The most common (nonantidepressant) medications used for anxiety are summarized in table 21.1.

Table 21.2. List of Sedative-Hypnotic Medications

Benzodiazepines		
Brand Name	**Chemical**	**Average Daily Dosage (mg/day)**
Dalmane	flurazepam	15–30
Restoril	temazepam	7.5–60
Halcion	triazolam	0.125–0.5
Other Sedative-Hypnotics		
Brand Name	**Chemical**	**Average Daily Dosage (mg/day)**
Noctec	chloral hydrate	500–2000
Ambien	Zolpidem	5–10
Eszopiclone	Lunesta	1–3
Antihistamines		
Brand Name	**Chemical**	**Average Daily Dosage (mg/day)**
Benadryl	diphenhydramine	25–300

REBOUND ACTIVITY

Some individuals, as the benzodiazepine level in their body declines, begin to experience an increase in anxiety called "rebound anxiety." In some cases, this anxiety can be quite severe and frightening. This is more common for the short-acting than long-acting drugs. If the person taking the benzodiazepine notices an increase in anxiety before the next dosage, the physician should be consulted. Sometimes the person will be switched from a short-acting to a long-acting benzodiazepine or buspirone to prevent rebound anxiety.

Sedative-Hypnotic Medications

Sedative-hypnotic drugs are used in the treatment of agitation and to facilitate sleep. Similar to antianxiety drugs, the most commonly used sedative-hypnotic drugs are benzodiazepines. A different type of sedative-hypnotic drugs is chloral hydrate. Antihistamines are also used sometimes as sedative-hypnotic drugs. The most common types of these drugs are listed in table 21.2.

SIDE EFFECTS OF ANTIANXIETY AND SEDATIVE-HYPNOTIC DRUGS
The most common side effect of these drugs is sedation and fatigue (except Buspar). With the long-acting benzodiazepines, the sedation can persist for more than a day after the drug has been taken. Because of the sedating effects, the intake of alcohol should be limited to not more than one drink per week, and appropriate cautions should be exercised when driving. The benzodiazepines can also affect memory and other cognitive abilities.

Chapter 22 | Complementary Health Approaches

Section 22.1 | Complementary Therapies: Evidence and Risks

This section contains text excerpted from the following sources: Text in this section begins with excerpts from "Anxiety at a Glance," National Center for Complementary and Integrative Health (NCCIH), December 2018; Text beginning with the heading "Complementary Health Approaches: Advising Clients about Evidence and Risks" is excerpted from "Complementary Health Approaches: Advising Clients about Evidence and Risks," Substance Abuse and Mental Health Services Administration (SAMHSA), 2015. Reviewed August 2020.

Researchers are examining ways in which complementary and integrative approaches might reduce anxiety or help people cope with it. Some studies have focused on the anxiety that people experience in everyday life or during stressful situations, while others have focused on anxiety disorders.

WHAT THE SCIENCE SAYS

Some complementary health approaches may help to relieve anxiety during stressful situations, such as medical procedures. Less is known about whether complementary health approaches can help to manage anxiety disorders.

Mind and Body Practices

- Relaxation techniques may reduce anxiety in people with chronic medical problems and those who are having medical procedures. However, cognitive-behavioral therapy (CBT) (a type of psychotherapy) may be more helpful than relaxation techniques in treating at least some types of anxiety disorders.
- Although some studies suggest that acupuncture might reduce anxiety, the research is too limited to allow definite conclusions to be reached.
- Hypnosis has been studied for anxiety related to medical or dental procedures. Some studies have had promising results, but the overall evidence is not conclusive.
- In some studies in people with cancer or other medical conditions, massage therapy helped to reduce anxiety; however, other studies did not find a beneficial effect.

Little research has been done on massage for anxiety disorders, and the studies that have been done have had conflicting results.

- Studies have looked at the effects of interventions involving mindfulness meditation on anxiety in various groups of people, including cancer patients, people with other chronic diseases, family caregivers, pregnant women, healthcare providers, employees, and students. Many but not all of these studies indicated that mindfulness was helpful for anxiety. There is some evidence that Transcendental Meditation may have a beneficial effect on anxiety. There has not been enough research to know whether mindfulness or other types of meditation are helpful for anxiety disorders.
- There is evidence that listening to music can reduce anxiety during illness or medical treatment.
- Studies suggest that meditative movement therapies (tai chi, qi gong, or yoga) might reduce anxiety, but the research is too limited to allow definite conclusions to be reached.
- Reiki and therapeutic touch have not been shown to be helpful for anxiety.

Natural Products

- Two studies, both supported by the National Center for Complementary and Integrative Health (NCCIH), suggest that a chamomile extract might be helpful in managing generalized anxiety disorder (GAD), but the studies are preliminary, and their findings are not conclusive.
- Kava may have a beneficial effect on anxiety. However, the use of kava supplements has been linked to a risk of severe liver damage.
- Melatonin has been studied as a possible alternative to conventional anxiety-reducing drugs for patients who are about to have surgery, and the results have been promising.
- There is not enough evidence on passionflower or valerian for anxiety to allow any conclusions to be reached.

Other Complementary Approaches

- Aromatherapy and homeopathy have not been shown to be helpful for anxiety.

SIDE EFFECTS AND RISKS

- Mind and body practices are generally safe for healthy people if properly performed by a qualified practitioner or taught by a well-trained instructor. As with any physical activity, practices that involve movement, such as yoga, pose some risk of injury. People with health conditions and pregnant women should talk with their healthcare providers about any mind and body practices they are considering and may need to modify or avoid some of them.
- Dietary supplements may have side effects and interact with medications.

COMPLEMENTARY HEALTH APPROACHES: ADVISING CLIENTS ABOUT EVIDENCE AND RISKS

Many clients receiving conventional evidence-based treatment for mental or substance-use disorders (SUDs) may also try various nonmainstream or complementary, health approaches to treat their disorders or to relieve symptoms; some may do so without professional guidance. Clients may also independently turn to complementary products or practices to address co-occurring medical issues such as pain or to achieve personal-health and wellness goals, such as weight loss. At the same time, an increasing number of medical facilities and behavioral health programs are including complementary health approaches in their menu of services.

Complementary therapies vary in their safety, cost, and evidence of effectiveness. Clients may spend a great deal of time and money on products and services without knowing whether or how they work. In addition, clients may be unaware that some complementary therapies can have side effects or adversely interact with medications.

Some clients may not tell their behavioral health service practitioners of their use of complementary therapies; other clients may ask practitioners whether complementary health approaches are helpful. Practitioners may also be called on to explain the benefits of any complementary practices offered by their treatment programs. This Advisory gives behavioral health service practitioners a brief overview of complementary health approaches and information on efficacy and cautions so that they can talk knowledgeably with clients and offer appropriate guidance.

WHAT ARE COMPLEMENTARY HEALTH APPROACHES?

The term "complementary health approaches" encompasses a group of diverse medical and healthcare systems, practices, and products that are not generally considered to be part of conventional medicine. Also called "mainstream," "modern," or "Western" medicine, conventional medicine is practiced by doctors holding medical degrees and by allied health professionals, and its practices are evaluated scientifically for evidence of effectiveness.

Most Americans use nonmainstream practices as complements, rather than as alternatives, to conventional medicine. Generally speaking, complementary therapies have not been evaluated as extensively and rigorously as practices in conventional medicine.

Many complementary therapies have emerged out of ancient medical systems such as Ayurvedic medicine from India, traditional Chinese medicine (which includes acupuncture), traditional African medicine, shamanism, and Native American healing practices. Other systems that offer complementary therapies, such as homeopathy and naturopathy, stem from practices that emerged in Europe beginning in the late 18th century.

An increasing number of medical care and behavioral health facilities now offer integrative health (also known as "integrative medicine"), which combines complementary practices with conventional treatment plans. More than 60 academic health centers and affiliate institutions in the United States, Canada, and Mexico are members of the Academic Consortium for Integrative Medicine and Health and include complementary health approaches in their curricula. According to the Consortium, integrative medicine and health "reaffirms the importance of the relationship between practitioner and patient, focuses on the whole person, is informed by evidence, and makes use of all appropriate therapeutic and lifestyle approaches, healthcare professionals and disciplines to achieve optimal health and healing."

Development of scientific evidence in the field of complementary and integrative medicine has been advanced by the National Institutes of Health's (NIH) National Center for Complementary and Integrative Health (NCCIH),* which funds and conducts research and provides information for consumers and practitioners. Some complementary therapies are now covered by health insurance or other reimbursement systems.

* On December 16, 2014, legislation was enacted that changed the name of the National Center for Complementary and Alternative Medicine (NCCAM) to the National Center
for Complementary and Integrative Health.

Section 22.2 | Anxiety and Complementary Health Approaches: What the Science Says

This section includes text excerpted from "Anxiety and Complementary Health Approaches: What the Science Says," National Center for Complementary and Integrative Health (NCCIH), August 2018.

MIND AND BODY APPROACHES
Acupuncture
Although some studies of acupuncture for anxiety have had positive outcomes, in general, many of the studies on acupuncture for anxiety have been of poor methodological quality or not of statistical significance. In addition, because the research is extremely variable (e.g., number and variety of acupuncture points, frequency of sessions, and duration of treatment), it is difficult to draw firm conclusions about potential benefits.

WHAT DOES THE RESEARCH SHOW?
- A 2012 review of 32 studies of acupuncture for anxiety found that although there have been some positive outcomes, the generally poor methodological quality,

combined with the wide range of outcome measures used, number and variety of points, frequency of sessions, and duration of treatment makes drawing firm conclusions difficult.

- A 2014 meta-analysis of 14 studies involving 1,034 participants on the efficacy of acupuncture in reducing preoperative anxiety found that acupuncture has a statistically significant effect relative to placebo or nontreatment controls, but the sample size was small. The meta-analysis supports the possibility that acupuncture is superior to placebo for preoperative anxiety.

SAFETY

- Acupuncture is generally considered safe when performed by an experienced practitioner using sterile needles. Reports of serious adverse events related to acupuncture are rare, but include infections and punctured organs.

Massage Therapy

In some studies massage therapy helped to reduce anxiety for people with cancer or other comorbid medical conditions; however, other studies did not find a statistically significant beneficial effect. Little research has been done on massage for anxiety disorders, and results have been conflicting.

WHAT DOES THE RESEARCH SHOW?

- A 2014 systematic review and meta-analysis of 18 randomized controlled trials involving 950 women with breast cancer did not find any significant effect of massage on anxiety.
- A 2013 randomized controlled trial of 60 cancer patients examined massage therapy for perioperative pain and anxiety in placement of vascular access devices and found that both massage therapy and structured attention proved beneficial for alleviating preoperative anxiety in these patients.

- A 2012 randomized trial involving 152 cardiac surgery patients found that massage therapy significantly reduced the pain, anxiety, and muscular tension and improved relaxation after cardiac surgery.
- Findings from a 2012 randomized controlled trial of 120 primiparous women with term pregnancy suggest that massage is an effective alternative intervention, decreasing pain and anxiety during labor.

SAFETY
- Massage therapy appears to have few risks if it is used appropriately and provided by a trained massage professional.

Mindfulness Meditation

Meditation therapy is commonly used and has been shown to be of small to modest benefit for people with anxiety-related symptoms. There is some evidence that Transcendental Meditation (TM) may have a beneficial effect on anxiety. However, there is a lack of studies with adequate statistical power in patients with clinically diagnosed anxiety disorders, which makes it difficult to draw firm conclusions about its efficacy for anxiety disorders.

WHAT DOES THE RESEARCH SHOW?
- A 2017 randomized controlled trial involving 57 participants with generalized anxiety disorder (GAD) found that mindfulness meditation training was associated with a significantly greater decrease in partial work days and decrease in healthcare utilization.
- A 2014 systematic review and meta-analysis of 47 trials with 3,515 participants found that mindfulness meditation programs had moderate evidence of improved anxiety. The reviewers concluded that clinicians should be aware that meditation programs can result in mild-to-moderate reductions of multiple negative dimensions of psychological stress.

- A 2012 systematic review and meta-analysis of 36 randomized controlled trials found evidence of some efficacy of meditative therapies in reducing anxiety symptoms; however, most studies included in the analysis measured only improvement in anxiety symptoms, but not anxiety disorders as clinically diagnosed.
- A 2006 Cochrane review of two randomized controlled trials concluded that because of the small number of studies, conclusions could not be drawn about the efficacy of meditation therapy for anxiety disorders.

SAFETY
- Meditation is generally considered to be safe for healthy people. However, people with physical limitations may not be able to participate in certain meditative practices involving movement.

Relaxation Techniques
Relaxation techniques may reduce anxiety in individuals with chronic medical problems and those who are having medical procedures. However, research demonstrates that conventional psychotherapy, for individuals with GAD, may be more effective than relaxation techniques.

WHAT DOES THE RESEARCH SHOW?
- A 2014 meta-analysis of a total of 41 studies involving 2,132 participants with generalized anxiety disorder found some indications that cognitive-behavioral therapy (CBT) was more effective than relaxation techniques over the long term.
- A 2016 randomized trial of 236 women undergoing large core breast biopsy found that adjunctive self-hypnotic relaxation decreased procedural pain and anxiety.
- A 2012 randomized controlled trial of 39 participants with inflammatory bowel disease (IBD) found that those who received the relaxation-training intervention showed a

statistically significant improvement in anxiety levels as compared to the control group.

SAFETY

- Relaxation techniques are generally considered safe for healthy people. People with serious physical- or mental-health problems should discuss relaxation techniques with their healthcare providers.

Natural Products
CHAMOMILE

There is some research that suggests that a chamomile extract may be helpful for generalized anxiety disorder, but the studies are preliminary, and their findings are not conclusive.

What Does the Research Show?

- A 2016 randomized controlled trial involving 179 participants with moderate-to-severe GAD found that chamomile extract produced a clinical meaningful reduction in anxiety symptoms over eight weeks.
- Results from a 2009 randomized, double-blind, placebo-controlled efficacy and tolerability trial of chamomile extract in 57 patients with mild-to-moderate GAD suggest that chamomile may have modest anxiolytic activity in patients with mild-to-moderate generalized anxiety disorder.

Safety

- There have been reports of allergic reactions, including rare cases of anaphylaxis, in people who have consumed or come into contact with chamomile products.
- People are more likely to experience allergic reactions to chamomile if they are allergic to related plants such as ragweed, chrysanthemums, marigolds, or daisies.
- Interactions between chamomile and cyclosporine and warfarin have been reported, and there are theoretical

reasons to suspect that chamomile might interact with other drugs as well.

KAVA

Kava extract may produce moderately beneficial effects on anxiety symptoms; however, the use of kava supplements has been linked to a risk of severe liver damage.

What Does the Research Show?

- A 2013 randomized controlled trial involving 75 participants with GAD concluded that standardized kava extract may be a moderately effective short-term option for the treatment of GAD.
- A 2011 review of 66 studies of herbal medicine for depression, anxiety, and insomnia found some evidence that kava may produce beneficial effects for anxiety disorders.
- A 2003 Cochrane review of 12 randomized controlled trials found that compared with placebo, kava extract may be an effective symptomatic treatment for anxiety, although the effect size appears small.

Safety

- The use of kava supplements has been linked to a risk of severe liver damage, according to the U.S. Food and Drug Administration (FDA).
- Kava has been associated with several cases of dystonia and may interact with several drugs, including drugs used for Parkinson disease (PD).
- However, a 2013 randomized controlled trial of 75 participants who received kava extract over a 6-week period found no significant differences across groups for liver function tests, nor any significant adverse reactions associated with kava administration. Long-term safety studies of kava are needed.

MELATONIN

There is some research that suggests melatonin may help reduce anxiety in patients who are about to have surgery and may be as effective as standard treatment with midazolam in reducing pre-operative anxiety.

What Does the Research Show?

- A 2017 randomized trial involving 80 children undergoing surgery found that melatonin was as effective as midazolam in reducing children's anxiety in both the preoperative room and at induction of anesthesia.
- A 2015 Cochrane review of 12 studies involving 774 participants found that melatonin compared to placebo, given as premedication, reduced preoperative anxiety (measured 50 to 100 minutes after administration) and may reduce postoperative anxiety (6 hours after surgery). The reviewers also found that melatonin may be equally as effective as standard treatment with midazolam in reducing preoperative anxiety.

Safety

- Melatonin supplements appear to be safe when used short term; less is known about long-term safety.

LAVENDER

Although some studies of lavender preparations for anxiety have shown some therapeutic effects, in general, many of these studies have been of poor methodological quality.

What Does the Research Show?

- A 2017 meta-analysis of five studies involving 1,165 participants with anxiety diagnoses found Silexan (lavender oil) to be significantly superior to placebo in ameliorating anxiety symptoms independently of diagnosis. The study also found a tendency for greater clinical effect when analyzing separately GAD patients in comparison with all other diagnosis.

- A 2012 systematic review of 15 randomized controlled trials concluded that methodological issues limit the extent to which any conclusions can be drawn regarding the efficacy of lavender for anxiety.

Safety

- When lavender teas and extracts are taken by mouth, they may cause headache, changes in appetite, and constipation.
- Using lavender supplements with sedative medications may increase drowsiness.

Section 22.3 | Relaxation Techniques

This section contains text excerpted from the following sources: Text under the heading "What Are Relaxation Techniques?" is excerpted from "Relaxation Techniques for Health," National Center for Complementary and Integrative Health (NCCIH), May 2016. Reviewed August 2020; Text under the heading "Relaxation Techniques for Stress" is excerpted from "5 Things To Know about Relaxation Techniques for Stress," National Center for Complementary and Integrative Health (NCCIH), August 3, 2020; Text under the heading "The Sigh Breath—the 'Instant Tranquillizer'" is excerpted from "Breath Work Techniques for Relaxation," U.S. Department of Veterans Affairs (VA), February 1, 2001. Reviewed August 2020; Text under the heading "Relaxation Exercise: Deep Breathing" is excerpted from "Relaxation Exercise: Deep Breathing," U.S. Department of Veterans Affairs (VA), September 2, 2015. Reviewed August 2020.

WHAT ARE RELAXATION TECHNIQUES?

Relaxation techniques include a number of practices such as progressive relaxation, guided imagery, biofeedback, self-hypnosis, and deep breathing exercises. The goal is similar in all: to produce the body's natural relaxation response, characterized by slower breathing, lower blood pressure, and a feeling of increased well-being.

Meditation and practices that include meditation with movement, such as yoga and tai chi, can also promote relaxation.

Stress management programs commonly include relaxation techniques. Relaxation techniques have also been studied to see whether they might be of value in managing various health problems.

RELAXATION TECHNIQUES FOR STRESS

In contrast to the stress response, the relaxation response slows the heart rate, lowers blood pressure, and decreases oxygen consumption and levels of stress hormones. In theory, voluntarily creating the relaxation response through regular use of relaxation techniques could counteract the negative effects of stress.

- Relaxation techniques are generally safe, but there is limited evidence of usefulness for specific health conditions. Research is under way to find out more about relaxation and health outcomes.
- Relaxation techniques often combine breathing and focused attention to calm the mind and the body. These techniques may be most effective when practiced regularly and combined with good nutrition, regular exercise, and a strong social support system.
- Most relaxation techniques can be self-taught and self-administered. Most methods require only brief instruction from a book or experienced practitioner before they can be done without assistance.
- Do not use relaxation techniques as a replacement for conventional care or to postpone seeing a doctor about a medical problem. Talk to your healthcare providers if you are considering using a relaxation technique for a particular health condition. This will help ensure coordinated and safe care.

THE SIGH BREATH—THE 'INSTANT TRANQUILLIZER'

The Sigh Breath is a very simple breathing method for releasing tension in your chest, diaphragm and neck areas.

It can be an excellent way of managing the symptoms of anxiety or panic. It is a moderate (rather than very deep) inhale through the nose followed by a fairly prolonged and slow exhale through the nose or mouth—as a prelude to allowing your breathing to become slower and shallower.

How to Use the Sigh Breath

- Mentally think or say to yourself "Stop!"
- Now breathe in through nose slowly and evenly. Pausing for just a second let the air out quite slowly through your nose. Remember that the inhale is a moderate, rather than a very deep in-breath. The out-breath is the key to the method. Be sure to prolong it. L-e-n-g-t-h-e-n your exhale. This helps retain carbon dioxide—your "natural tranquilizer."
- As you let the air out let go! Relax your muscles—release as much tension as you can. Pay particular attention to the muscles in your face, jaw, shoulders, and abdomen.
- Pay attention to the natural pause that occurs at the end of the exhale. No need to think about breathing in—this will happen naturally after a second or two. Simply enjoy this moment of stillness between breathing cycles.
- As the in-breath begins, direct your attention outside yourself to what is happening in the outside world—"See Clearly—Hear Clearly." Silently pay attention to what you can see and hear without listing or naming anything.

Although the method involves five steps, the whole cycle of in-breath—brief pause—out-breath takes only a few seconds.

The Sigh Breath is a way of interrupting the buildup of physical stress and tension rather than a breathing technique to do over and over again. Initially one or two Sigh Breaths every half hour or so may be appropriate. Then aim to reduce the need to do it except for very tense periods.

Why Use the Sigh Breath?

- It instantly reduces your tension level through temporarily raising your blood carbon dioxide level.
- The "See Clearly—Hear Clearly" part of the method directs your attention outside of yourself. This interrupts the common and unuseful tendency that most of us have, when we feel anxious or upset, to ruminate—to become very absorbed with our thoughts and feelings.

- It engages your attention for a few moments. When you use it regularly you momentarily interrupt your internal stress-building loop—the loop in which your stressful thoughts result in stressful feelings which, in turn, exacerbate the stressful thoughts of negative thoughts—negative feelings—negative thoughts. This technique takes you out of the loop and into practical action.
- It helps draw your attention to the buildup of physical tension in your body—and especially in the throat, chest, and abdomen.
- It gives you something to do when you feel anxious or panicky, rather than simply remain a passive victim of your reaction to a situation.
- It makes you aware of and interrupts the common tendency to hold or restrict your breath when anxious.

EASY BREATHING

Maintaining an easy breathing pattern, where your chest and diaphragm are relaxed and moving naturally in harmony with each inhale and exhale helps redevelop and maintain a comfortable physical state with a clear and alert mind.

(In the beginning it is likely that accumulated tensions and poor breathing habits may have produced an uneven breathing pattern. If this is the case you may find it helpful to first use the Sigh Breath method a few times to begin calming and stabilizing your breathing.)

How to Use Easy Breathing

- Pay attention to the natural, effortless movement of your breathing cycle. Feel the movements and sensations.
- Pay attention to the inhale, then the slight pause, followed by the natural exhale, and then another slight pause.
- Aim to have your breathing become shallower and slower. Do not force this otherwise it will have the opposite effect. The slowing down should occur gradually and gently.
- Do this for three to ten minutes—paying attention to nothing else.

Through practice you may discover ways of utilizing Easy Breathing as a quick relaxer—a way of relaxing quickly for a few moments. As you experiment with the different breathing methods aim to discover which methods work best for you in different situations in your life.

When to Use Easy Breathing

- Whenever you wish to pace yourself and maintain a calmer and more centered internal state—at work, in sport, socially, etc.
- When you wish to clear your thinking in order to give your full attention to an important matter.
- As a quick relaxer—especially when it is inappropriate to relax with eyes closed, or to fully stop what you are doing.
- To develop the habit of maintaining a clear mind and calm body. Use Easy Breathing in odd spare moments: in elevators, in waiting lines, in waiting rooms, at traffic lights, during the commercial breaks when watching TV, while listening to someone, waiting on the phone, or when you are being delayed. In this way you can turn what might have otherwise been a frustrating or irritating event into a beneficial and centering experience.
- To develop an ongoing natural awareness of your physical state—so that any chest tightness or breathing unevenness alerts you to take action to clear your thinking and calm your body.
- To train yourself to feel mentally and physically comfortable even when under pressure.

Benefits of Easy Breathing

- Helps defuse the physical effects of the stress response.
- Provides an instant break and reduces frantic mental activity by centering your attention on a single issue rather than having it scattered.
- Gradually builds up your depleted store of carbon dioxide—your natural tranquilizer.

- Enables you to take a mental and physical break without stopping what you are doing.
- Enables you to maintain physical comfort while being mentally active.

RELAXATION EXERCISE: DEEP BREATHING

Deep breathing is a good way to relax. We do not always remember to breathe deeply. Most adults breathe from the chest, which is known as "shallow breathing." When you breathe deeply, your body takes in more oxygen. You exhale more carbon dioxide. Your body naturally "resets" itself to a more relaxed and calm state.

Deep breathing can be useful for anyone who has stress. You can practice deep breathing during your workday when you are feeling stressed or anxious. And you can choose to take a couple minutes and breathe deeply each day, or just use it when you need it.

Deep breathing does not just work for handling day-to-day stress. It can be especially helpful to Veterans and civilians who have experienced traumatic events (such as military combat or a civilian assault). Deep breathing can help you cope with the stress from these events. Symptoms, such as anxiety, "panic" or feeling "stuck in alarm mode" often respond well to deep breathing.

Deep Breathing

This exercise only takes a few minutes and can be performed anywhere. Nobody has to know you are doing it.

You may do this exercise with your eyes open or closed. If you have gone through traumatic stress you may find that keeping eyes open helps you to stay "grounded" in the "here and now." Do what is most comfortable for you.

Here is how to do it:

- Sit comfortably or lie down.
- Place one hand on your stomach and one hand on your chest.
- Breathe in slowly through your nose.
- Feel your stomach expand as you inhale. If you are breathing from the stomach, the hand on your chest should not move.

- Focus on filling up your lower lungs with air.
- Slowly exhale, releasing all the air out through your mouth.
- Use your hand to feel your stomach fall as you exhale.
- Practice breathing four to six breaths per minute (about one full inhale and exhale per 10 to 15 seconds).
- Repeat this up to ten times.

If you begin to get light headed, return to your normal breathing. Try deep breathing now and notice the difference it can make.

Section 22.4 | Mindfulness Practice in the Treatment of Anxiety

This section includes text excerpted from "Mindfulness Practice in the Treatment of Traumatic Stress," National Center for Posttraumatic Stress Disorder (NCPTSD), U.S. Department of Veterans Affairs (VA), January 13, 2020.

WHAT IS MINDFULNESS?

Mindfulness is a way of thinking and focusing that can help you become more aware of your present experiences. Practicing mindfulness can be as simple as noticing the taste of a mint on your tongue. There are some things you might do every day without even thinking about them, such as brushing your teeth in the morning. Mindfulness involves paying attention to the feelings and sensations of these experiences.

While researchers have not yet studied the effects of mindfulness practice in helping trauma survivors diagnosed with posttraumatic stress disorder (PTSD), research has shown mindfulness to be helpful with other anxiety problems. It has also been shown to help with symptoms of PTSD, such as avoidance and hyperarousal. If you have gone through trauma, you may want to learn what mindfulness is and how it might be helpful to you.

Mindfulness practice has two key parts:
- Paying attention to and being aware of the present moment
- Accepting or being willing to experience your thoughts and feelings without judging them

For example, focusing on the inhale and exhale of your breathing is one way to concentrate on the present moment. Mindfulness involves allowing your thoughts and feelings to pass without either clinging to them or pushing them away. You just let them take their natural course. While practicing mindfulness, you may become distracted by your thoughts and that is okay. The process is about being willing to notice where your thoughts take you, and then bringing your attention back to the present.

HOW CAN MINDFULNESS HELP REDUCE TRAUMA REACTIONS?

Mindfulness might increase your ability to cope with difficult emotions, such as anxiety and depression. Practicing mindfulness can help you to be more focused and aware of the present moment while also being more willing to experience the difficult emotions that sometimes come up after trauma. For example, mindfulness practice might help you to notice your thoughts and feelings more and to be able to just let them go, without labeling them as "good" or "bad" and without acting on them by avoiding or behaving impulsively.

Mindfulness is a practice, a continual process. Although it may be hard to do at first, regular mindfulness practice can help you notice your thoughts and learn to take a step back from them. Mindfulness practice can also help you develop more compassion toward yourself and others. You may be less likely to sit in judgment of your thoughts, feelings, and actions. You may become less critical of yourself. Using mindfulness can help you become more aware and gentle in response to your trauma reactions. This is an important step in recovery.

Cognitive processing therapy (CPT) and prolonged exposure (PE) have been shown to be the most effective treatments for PTSD. In both of these treatments, you are asked to write or talk about trauma with the guidance of your therapist. Mindfulness can prepare you for these treatments by giving you skills and confidence that you can handle your feelings. As you learn to be mindful, you learn to observe what is happening in your body and your mind. You can learn to be more willing to cope with difficult thoughts and feelings in a healthy way. This will help you keep going when you are asked to think and talk about your trauma in treatment. In this way you may get even more out of the PTSD treatment.

There are several types of therapy that use mindfulness practices. These therapies have been used to treat problems that often affect people with PTSD, such as anxiety, depression, and substance use. The therapies may target specific problems such as:

- Difficult feelings and stress in daily living
- The stress of physical health problems, such as chronic pain
- Negative thinking patterns that can lead to repeated episodes of depression
- Trouble working towards your goals in life
- Urges to use drugs or alcohol

SUMMING IT UP

Mindfulness practices may be of benefit to trauma survivors. Research findings show that mindfulness can help with problems and symptoms often experienced by survivors. Mindfulness could be used by itself or together with standard treatments proven effective for PTSD.

MINDFULNESS COACH APP

Also see the Mindfulness Coach App. Grounding yourself in the present moment can help you cope better with unpleasant thoughts and emotions. The Mindfulness Coach app will help you do this.

Section 22.5 | Abdominal Breathing

This section includes text excerpted from "Abdominal Breathing," Mental Illness Research, Education and Clinical Centers (MIRECC), U.S. Department of Veterans Affairs (VA), July 2013. Reviewed August 2020.

WHAT IS ABDOMINAL BREATHING?

The goal of breath-focused relaxation is to shift from quick, shallow chest breathing to deeper, more relaxed abdominal breathing.

During times of stress, our natural tendency is to either hold our breath, or to breathe in a shallow, rapid manner. When we are relaxed our breathing is naturally slower and deeper. When stress is chronic, we may habitually breathe shallowly, never really discharging the stale air from our lungs. Holding in your stomach for reasons of vanity also restricts breathing. In order to take a full deep breath, we must allow our diaphragm (the muscle separating our chest cavity from the abdominal cavity below the lungs) to drop down and our abdomen to expand. If we keep our stomach muscles held in tight when we breathe, we restrict the expansion of our lungs and rob our bodies of optimal oxygen. This puts our bodies in a state of alarm that creates the sensation of anxiety. Taking a few slow, deep breaths sends the signal to our body to relax. Deep breathing is also referred to as "abdominal breathing," "disphragmatic breathing," or "belly breathing." Abdominal breathing is a form of relaxation that you can use any time to help you to calm yourself physically and mentally and in turn, decrease stress.

INSTRUCTIONS FOR LEARNING ABDOMINAL BREATHING

- Place one hand, palm side down, on your chest. Place the other hand, palm side down, on your stomach.
- Breathe in through your nose to a slow count of 3 or 4 (one ...two ...three... four...). Notice the motion of each hand. When you breathe in, does the hand on your chest move? If so, which way does it move (out/up or in/down) and how much does it move? Does the hand on your stomach move? If so, which way (out or in) and how much?
- Now exhale through your nose, again to a slow count of 3 or 4. Notice again how each of your hands moves.

For the most relaxing breath, the hand on your chest should move very little while the hand on your stomach pushes out significantly on the inhale (in-breath) and goes back in on the exhale (out breath). A common problem is for the chest to inflate on the in-breath while the stomach stays still or even sucks in. When this happens, only the upper part of the lungs (the part behind the upper chest) is being used. When a full deep breath is properly taken, the diaphragm muscle drops down into the abdominal cavity to make room for the lungs to expand. As the diaphragm muscle drops down, it pushes the organs in the abdomen forward to make more room for the lungs. That is why the stomach goes out when you take the most relaxing type of breath.

Learning to take abdominal breaths versus chest breathing is a challenge for some people. The following tips can make it easier:

- Imagine yourself filling a medium-sized balloon in your stomach each time you inhale and releasing the air in the balloon when you exhale.
- Breathe in the same amount of air you breathe out.
- It is sometimes easier to first learn abdominal breathing while lying on your back with your hand on your stomach. It is easier to feel the stomach motion in this position versus sitting or standing.
- It is best to only practice a few deep breaths at a time at first. This is because deep breathing can make you feel light-headed if you are not used to it. If you begin to feel light headed, it is just your body's signal that it has had enough practice for now. Return to your normal breathing and practice again later. With practice, you will be able to take a greater number of deep breaths without becoming light-headed.
- Start practicing this deep breathing technique when you are calm so you have mastered it and are ready to use it when you are stressed.

KEY POINTS

- Abdominal breathing can help you achieve a state of relaxation because it has both meditative (mentally calming) and sedating (physically calming) qualities.
- Try not to get frustrated by "worry" or "to-do" thoughts that enter your head while you are relaxing. Gently let these thoughts pass and return to the task at hand. Focusing on your deep breathing will help you. Sometimes, it also helps to "place" busy thoughts on

an imaginary conveyor belt such as those found at the airport—eventually your thought luggage will come back round where you can pick it up after your relaxation trip. Or, mentally set your concerns on a shelf until you are ready to address them.

- Practice this type of breathing for about five minutes, one or more times a day, most days of the week.
- Learning to focus on one of the most calming processes in the body, namely your breathing, is one of the most reliable ways to achieve a relaxed state!
- This is a great relaxation exercise to learn because you can do it anywhere, anytime you want to take the edge off your anxiety stress level.
- It is normal for this new method of breathing to feel awkward at first. With practice it will feel more natural.

LONGER RELAXATION EXERCISES

Deep breathing can be expanded into a longer relaxation exercise as well. Two examples are given below:

Three-Part Rhythmic Breathing

Inhale... hold the breath... and then exhale... with the inhale, hold, and exhale each being of equal length. Inhale and exhale completely using the entire length of the lungs. Keep your shoulders and face relaxed while you hold your breath. Use a count that is comfortable for you. Repeat five times.

Breathing with Imagery

For about 30 seconds, simply relax with your eyes closed. Then start to pay attention to your breathing. Let your breathing become slow and relaxed, like a person sleeping. Feel the air entering through your nose with each inhalation, and feel your breath leave as you exhale. Imagine the tension leaving your body with each breath.

Now imagine that, as you breathe in, the air comes into your nose and caresses your face like a gentle breeze. As you breathe out, the exhalation carries away the tension from your face. As you breathe slowly in and out, tension gradually leaves your body and you become more and more relaxed.

Now imagine that, as you breathe in, the gentle air enters your nose and spreads relaxation up over the top of your head. As you exhale, imagine the tension leaving this area and passing out of our body. Then imagine the next breath carrying relaxation over your face, your scalp, and both sides of your head. As you exhale, let any tension flow out easily.

If other thoughts come to mind, simply return to paying attention to your breathing. Your breathing is slow and easy, with no effort at all. Let your body relax.

Now let your breath carry relaxation to your neck. As you exhale, tension passes out of your neck and out of your body with the exhaled air. Feel a breath carry relaxation into your shoulders. As you exhale, any tension leaves your shoulders and passes out of your body.

Now one breath at a time, focus your attention on each part of your body from the top down: your upper arms, forearms, hands, chest, back, stomach, hips, thighs, knees, calves, ankles, and feet. Imagine each breath of air carrying relaxation into each part of your body. As you breathe out, let any tension pass out through your nostrils.

This exercise takes several minutes. Do it at your own pace. When you have finished, sit quietly for a minute or two more.

Section 22.6 | Meditative Movement Therapies: Yoga, Tai Chi, and Qi Gong

This section contains text excerpted from the following sources: Text beginning with the heading "Yoga for Children and Adolescents" is excerpted from "Yoga for Health: What the Science Says," National Center for Complementary and Integrative Health (NCCIH), February 2020; Text under the heading "What Are Tai Chi and Qi Gong?" is excerpted from "Whole Health: Information for Veterans," U.S. Department of Veterans Affairs (VA), July 13, 2018; Text under the heading "Tai Chi: A Modern Take on an Ancient Practice" is excerpted from "Tai Chi and Your Health," *NIH News in Health*, National Institutes of Health (NIH), December 2016. Reviewed August 2020; Text under the heading "What You Should Know about Tai Chi for Health" is excerpted from "5 Tips: What You Should Know about Tai Chi for Health," National Center for Complementary and Integrative Health (NCCIH), August 3, 2020; Text under the heading "What Does the Research Show about Yoga, Tai Chi, and Qi Gong?" is excerpted from "Mind and Body Approaches for Stress and Anxiety: What the Science Says," National Center for Complementary and Integrative Health (NCCIH), April 2020.

YOGA FOR CHILDREN AND ADOLESCENTS

The American Academy of Pediatrics (AAP) recommends yoga as a safe and potentially effective therapy for children and adolescents coping with emotional, mental, physical, and behavioral health conditions. Yoga can help children learn to self-regulate, focus on the task at hand, and handle problems peacefully. Yoga may also improve balance, relieve tension, and increase strength when practiced regularly. Because some yoga poses are harder than others, the AAP cautions that even children who are flexible and in good shape should start slowly.

What Does the Research Show?

- A 2016 review found that school-based yoga programs seem to help improve adolescents' health.
- A 2015 systematic review of 16 studies (including 6 randomized controlled trials, 2 nonrandomized preintervention-postintervention control-group designs, 7 uncontrolled preintervention-postintervention studies, and 1 case study) for yoga interventions addressing anxiety among children and adolescents concluded that nearly all studies included in the review indicated reduced anxiety following a yoga intervention. However, the reviewers noted that because of the wide variety of study populations, limitations in some study designs, and

variable outcome measures, further research is needed to enhance the ability to generalize and apply yoga to reduce anxiety.

YOGA FOR OLDER ADULTS

Yoga's popularity among older Americans is growing. National survey data show that 6.7 percent of U.S. adults 65 years of age and over practiced yoga in 2017, as compared to 3.3 percent in 2012, 2 percent in 2007, and 1.3 percent in 2002.

Older adults who practice yoga should put safety first. It is a good idea to start with an appropriate yoga class—such as one called "gentle yoga" or "seniors yoga"—to get individualized advice and learn correct form. Chair yoga is an even gentler option for seniors with limited mobility. And it is important for older people with medical issues to talk to both their healthcare providers and the yoga teacher before starting yoga.

YOGA FOR HEALTH AND WELL-BEING

Only a small amount of research has investigated yoga for general well-being, such as improving sleep and reducing stress, and the findings have not been completely consistent. Nevertheless, some preliminary research results suggest that yoga may have several different types of benefits for general well-being.

What Does the Research Show?
- **Stress management.** Some research indicates that practicing yoga can lead to improvements in physical or psychological aspects of stress.
- **Balance.** Several studies that looked at the effect of yoga on balance in healthy people found evidence of improvements.
- **Positive mental health.** Some but not all studies that looked at the effects of yoga on positive aspects of mental health found evidence of benefits, such as better resilience or general mental well-being.

- **Health habits.** A survey of young adults showed that practicing yoga regularly was associated with better eating and physical activity habits, such as more servings of fruits and vegetables, fewer servings of sugar-sweetened beverages, and more hours of moderate-to-vigorous activity. But, it was not clear from this study whether yoga motivates people to practice better health habits or whether people with healthier habits are more likely to do yoga. In another study, however, in which previously inactive people were randomly assigned to participate or not participate in ten weeks of yoga classes, those who participated in yoga increased their total physical activity.
- **Quitting smoking.** Programs that include yoga have been evaluated to see whether they help people quit smoking. In most studies of this type, yoga reduced cigarette cravings and the number of cigarettes smoked. Findings suggest that yoga may be a helpful addition to smoking cessation programs.
- **Weight control.** In studies of yoga in people who were overweight or obese, practicing yoga has been associated with a reduction in body mass index (BMI). An NCCIH-supported comparison of different yoga-based programs for weight control showed that the most helpful programs had longer and more frequent yoga sessions, a longer duration of the overall program, a yoga-based dietary component, a residential component (such as a full weekend to start the program), inclusion of a larger number of elements of yoga, and home practice.

YOGA FOR ANXIETY OR DEPRESSION

Yoga may be helpful for anxiety or depressive symptoms associated with difficult life situations. However, the research on yoga for anxiety disorders, clinical depression, or posttraumatic stress disorder (PTSD), although mildly positive, is still very preliminary.

WHAT ARE TAI CHI AND QI GONG?

Tai chi and qi gong are mind-body practices that have been used for thousands of years to promote health. Tai chi is one form of qi gong, but there are some differences in how they are practiced. Both target the energy of the body, traditionally called "qi" (pronounced "chee"), via focused breath and movements.

Tai chi means "grand ultimate fist" in Chinese, and it has origins in various martial arts practices. Author of the *Harvard Medical School Guide to Tai Chi*, Dr. Peter Wayne, describes tai chi practice in terms of "eight active ingredients:"

- **Awareness.** Tai chi practice develops focus and mindful awareness.
- **Intention.** Tai chi practice actively uses images and visualization to enhance its health effects.
- **Structural integration.** Tai chi practice focuses on good posture and how a person positions the body. Good body positioning leads to better body function, and better function leads to better posture.
- **Active relaxation.** Tai chi practice is a form of moving meditation, using flowing and relaxing movements.
- **Strengthening and flexibility.** Tai chi uses slow movements that are done repetitively. Weight is shifted from leg-to-leg and different parts of the body are flexed and extended.
- **Natural, freer breathing.** Tai chi practice teaches breathing skills, leading to many health benefits.
- **Social support.** Tai chi practice can involve being a part of a group class. This allows people to form community.
- **Embodied spirituality.** Tai chi practice allows the body, mind, and spirit to work together which helps a person focus on how they connect with others around them.

The "eight active ingredients" described for tai chi also apply to qi gong. Like tai chi, qi gong uses simple movements, but it also focuses on increasing and improving the flow of qi. There are many other types of qi gong in addition to those that use movement. Qi gong translates as "cultivation of life energy," and in traditional Chinese medicine, "life energy" supports health and wellness.

The movements of qi gong are similar to tai chi in that they are slow, intentional, and coordinated with breath and/or focused attention. One difference is that qi gong postures are often performed standing in place or even while standing still.

TAI CHI: A MODERN TAKE ON AN ANCIENT PRACTICE

Tai chi is an ancient mind and body practice. While more research is needed, studies suggest that it may have many health benefits.

Tai chi is sometimes referred to as "moving meditation." There are many types of tai chi. They typically combine slow movements with breathing patterns and mental focus and relaxation. Movements may be done while walking, standing, or sitting.

"At its root, tai chi is about treating the whole person and enhancing the balance and crosstalk between the body's systems," says Dr. Peter Wayne, a longtime tai chi researcher at Harvard Medical School. "It is a promising intervention for preserving and improving many areas of health, especially in older adults."

Research suggests that practicing tai chi might help improve posture and confidence, how you think and manage emotions, and your quality of life. Studies have found that it may help people with fibromyalgia sleep better and cope with pain, fatigue, and depression. Regular practice may also improve quality of life and mood in people with chronic heart failure or cancer. Older adults may find that tai chi can help improve sleep quality and protect learning, memory, and other mental functions.

Further study will be needed to fully evaluate and confirm the potential benefits of tai chi. But since the practice involves moving slowly and mindfully, there is little chance of harm when done correctly.

"Whether you are interested in trying tai chi to help with a chronic health issue or the stresses of everyday life, tai chi—if taught properly—can be a great complement to other ways of healthy living and rehabilitation," Wayne says. "I think we are all looking for tools to help us live productive, long lives with a little more grace and ease."

WHAT YOU SHOULD KNOW ABOUT TAI CHI FOR HEALTH

- Research findings suggest that practicing tai chi may improve balance and stability in older people and reduce the risk of falls. There is also some evidence that tai chi may improve balance impairments in people with mild-to-moderate Parkinson disease.

- There is some evidence to suggest that practicing tai chi may help people manage chronic pain associated with knee osteoarthritis and help people with fibromyalgia sleep better and cope with pain, fatigue, and depression.

- Although tai chi has not been shown to have an effect on the disease activity of rheumatoid arthritis (e.g., tender and swollen joints, activities of daily living), there is some evidence that tai chi may improve lower extremity (ankle) range of motion in people with rheumatoid arthritis. It is not known if tai chi improves pain associated with rheumatoid arthritis or quality of life (QOL).

- Tai chi may promote QOL and mood in people with heart failure and cancer. Tai chi also may offer psychological benefits, such as reducing anxiety. However, differences in how the research on anxiety was conducted make it difficult to draw firm conclusions about this.

- Take charge of your health—talk with your healthcare providers about any complementary health approaches you use. Together, you can make shared, well-informed decisions.

WHAT DOES THE RESEARCH SHOW ABOUT YOGA, TAI CHI, AND QI GONG?

A range of research has examined the relationship between exercise and depression. Results from a much smaller body of research suggest that exercise may also affect stress and anxiety symptoms. Even less certain is the role of yoga, tai chi, and qi gong—for these and other psychological factors, but there is some limited evidence that yoga, as an adjunctive therapy, may be helpful for people with anxiety symptoms.

- **Yoga for children and adolescents.** A 2020 systematic review of 27 studies involving the effects of yoga on children and adolescents with varying health statuses found that in studies assessing anxiety and depression, 58 percent showed reductions in both symptoms, while 25 percent showed reductions in anxiety only. Additionally, 70 percent of studies included in the review that assessed anxiety alone showed improvements. However, the reviewers noted that the studies included in the review were of weak-to-moderate methodological quality.
- **Yoga, tai chi, and qi gong for anxiety.** A 2019 review concluded that yoga as an adjunctive therapy facilitates treatment of anxiety disorders, particularly panic disorder. The review also found that tai chi and qi gong may be helpful as adjunctive therapies for depression, but effects are inconsistent.
- **Yoga for anxiety.** A 2018 systematic review and meta-analysis of 8 studies of yoga for anxiety (involving 319 participants with anxiety disorders or elevated levels of anxiety) found evidence that yoga might have short-term benefits in reducing the intensity of anxiety. However, when only people with diagnosed anxiety disorders were included in the analysis, there was no benefit. In a 2013 systematic review of 23 studies (involving 1,722 participants) of yoga for anxiety associated with life situations, yoga seemed to be helpful in some instances but not others. In general, results were more favorable for interventions that included at least 10 yoga sessions. The studies were of medium to poor quality, so definite conclusions about yoga's effectiveness could not be reached.

Safety

- Yoga is generally considered a safe form of physical activity for healthy people when performed properly, under the guidance of a qualified instructor. However, as with other forms of physical activity, injuries can occur. The most common injuries are sprains and strains. Serious injuries are rare. The risk of injury associated with yoga is lower than that for higher impact physical activities.

- Older people may need to be particularly cautious when practicing yoga. The rate of yoga-related injuries treated in emergency departments (ED) is higher in people 65 years of age and older than in younger adults.

Section 22.7 | Massage Therapy

This section contains text excerpted from the following sources: Text beginning with the heading "What Is Massage Therapy Used For?" is excerpted from "Massage Therapy: What You Need To Know," National Center for Complementary and Integrative Health (NCCIH), May 2019; Text under the heading "What You Need to Know" is excerpted from "Massage Therapy," *NIH News in Health*, National Institutes of Health (NIH), July 2012. Reviewed August 2020.

WHAT IS MASSAGE THERAPY USED FOR?

Massage therapy is used to help manage a health condition or enhance wellness. It involves manipulating the soft tissues of the body. Massage has been practiced in most cultures, both Eastern and Western, throughout human history, and was one of the earliest tools that people used to try to relieve pain.

WHAT ARE THE DIFFERENT TYPES OF MASSAGE?

The term "massage therapy" includes many techniques. The most common form of massage therapy in Western countries is called "Swedish" or "classical massage;" it is the core of most massage training programs. Other styles include sports massage, clinical massage to accomplish specific goals such as releasing muscle spasms, and massage traditions derived from Eastern cultures, such as Shiatsu and Tuina.

CAN MASSAGE HELP CANCER PATIENTS?

With appropriate precautions, massage therapy can be part of supportive care for cancer patients who would like to try it; however, the evidence that it can relieve pain and anxiety is not strong.

- Massage therapy, with or without aromatherapy (the use of essential oils) has been used to attempt to relieve pain, anxiety, and other symptoms in people with cancer. A 2016 evaluation of 19 studies (more than 1,200 participants) of massage for cancer patients found some evidence that massage might help with pain and anxiety, but the quality of the evidence was very low (because most studies were small and some may have been biased), and findings were not consistent.
- Clinical practice guidelines (guidance for healthcare providers) for the care of breast cancer patients include massage as one of several approaches that may be helpful for stress reduction, anxiety, depression, fatigue, and quality of life. Clinical practice guidelines for the care of lung cancer patients suggest that massage therapy could be added as part of supportive care in patients whose anxiety or pain is not adequately controlled by usual care.
- Massage therapists may need to modify their usual techniques when working with cancer patients; for example, they may have to use less pressure than usual in areas that are sensitive because of cancer or cancer treatments.

CAN MASSAGE BE HELPFUL FOR FIBROMYALGIA SYMPTOMS?

Massage therapy may be helpful for some fibromyalgia symptoms if it is continued for long enough.

- A 2014 evaluation of 9 studies (404 total participants) concluded that massage therapy, if continued for at least 5 weeks, improved pain, anxiety, and depression in people with fibromyalgia but did not have an effect on sleep disturbance.

- A 2015 evaluation of 10 studies (478 total participants) compared the effects of different kinds of massage therapy and found that most styles of massage had beneficial effects on quality of life (QOL) in people with fibromyalgia. Swedish massage may be an exception; 2 studies of this type of massage (56 total participants) did not show benefits.

CAN MASSAGE THERAPY BE HELPFUL FOR PEOPLE WITH HUMAN IMMUNODEFICIENCY VIRUS AND ACQUIRED IMMUNODEFICIENCY SYNDROME?

There is some evidence that massage therapy may have benefits for anxiety, depression, and QOL in people with human immunodeficiency virus (HIV) and acquired immunodeficiency syndrome (AIDS), but the amount of research and number of people studied are small.

- Massage therapy may help improve the QOL for people with HIV or AIDS, a 2010 review of 4 studies with a total of 178 participants concluded.
- More recently, a 2013 study of 54 people indicated that massage may be helpful for depression in people with HIV, and a 2017 study of 29 people with HIV suggested that massage may be helpful for anxiety.

WHAT ARE THE RISKS OF MASSAGE THERAPY?

The risk of harmful effects from massage therapy appears to be low. However, there have been rare reports of serious side effects, such as a blood clot, nerve injury, or bone fracture. Some of the reported cases have involved vigorous types of massage, such as deep tissue massage, or patients who might be at increased risk of injury, such as elderly people.

WHAT YOU NEED TO KNOW

Many people associate massage with vacations or spas and consider them something of a luxury. But, research is beginning to suggest

this ancient form of hands-on healing may be more than an indul-
gence—may help improve your health.

Massage therapists use their fingers, hands, forearms, and
elbows to manipulate the muscles and other soft tissues of the body.
Variations in focus and technique lead to different types of massage,
including Swedish, deep tissue, and sports massage.

In Swedish massage, the focus is general and the therapist may
use long strokes, kneading, deep circular movements, vibration and
tapping. With a deep tissue massage, the focus is more targeted, as
therapists work on specific areas of concern or pain. These areas
may have muscle "knots" or places of tissue restriction.

Some common reasons for getting a massage are to relieve pain,
heal sports injuries, reduce stress, relax, ease anxiety or depression, and aid general wellness. Unfortunately, scientific evidence
on massage therapy is limited. Researchers are actively trying to
understand exactly how massage works, how much is best, and
how it might help with specific health conditions. Some positive
benefits have been reported.

"Massage therapy has been noted to relax the nervous system by
slowing heart rate and blood pressure. Stress and pain hormones are
also decreased by massage, reducing pain and enhancing immune
function," says Dr. Tiffany Field, who heads a touch research
institute at the University of Miami Medical School. Much of her
National Institutes of Health (NIH)-funded research focuses on
the importance of massage for pregnant women and infants. Some
of her studies suggest that massage may improve weight-gain and
immune system function in preterm infants.

A study published earlier this year looked at how massage affects
muscles at the molecular level. The findings suggest that kneading
eases sore muscles after exercise by turning off genes associated
with inflammation and turning on genes that help muscles heal.

An NIH-supported study found that an hour-long "dose" of
Swedish massage therapy once a week was optimal for knee pain
from osteoarthritis, especially when practical matters such as time,
labor, and convenience were considered. Other research suggests
that massage therapy is effective in reducing and managing chronic
low-back pain, which affects millions of Americans.

Section 22.8 | **Chamomile: Is It an Effective Herbal Supplement?**

This section includes text excerpted from "Chamomile," National Center for Complementary and Integrative Health (NCCIH), May 2020.

- There are two types of chamomile: German chamomile and Roman chamomile. This section focuses on German chamomile.
- Chamomile was described in ancient medical writings and was an important medicinal herb in ancient Egypt, Greece, and Rome.
- Today, chamomile is promoted for sleeplessness, anxiety, and gastrointestinal conditions, such as upset stomach, gas, and diarrhea. It is also used topically for skin conditions and for mouth sores resulting from cancer treatment.

HOW MUCH DO WE KNOW?
- Not much is known about the health effects of chamomile because there are few studies on chamomile in people for individual conditions. Also, some studies look at products made of chamomile plus other herbs, so it is difficult to know chamomile's role from those studies.

WHAT HAVE WE LEARNED?
- Some preliminary studies suggest that a chamomile dietary supplement might be helpful for generalized anxiety disorder (GAD).
- Some research has found that products containing certain combinations of herbs that include chamomile may be of benefit for upset stomach, for diarrhea in children, and for infants with colic. But, chamomile alone has not been shown to be helpful for these conditions.
- There is very little information on chamomile's effect on insomnia. A 2019 review of six small studies included only one study on insomnia. That one study found

that chamomile had no benefit for insomnia. The same 2019 review looked at five studies on chamomile's effect in noninsomnia populations. The review concluded that chamomile might help improve the individual component of sleep quality over a 4-week period in people without insomnia.

WHAT DO WE KNOW ABOUT SAFETY?

- Chamomile is likely safe when used in amounts commonly found in teas. It might be safe when used orally for medicinal purposes over the short term. The long-term safety of using chamomile on the skin for medicinal purposes is unknown.
- Side effects are uncommon and may include nausea, dizziness, and allergic reactions. Rare cases of anaphylaxis (a life-threatening allergic reaction) have occurred in people who consumed or came into contact with chamomile products.
- People are more likely to experience allergic reactions to chamomile if they are allergic to related plants such as ragweed, chrysanthemums, marigolds, or daisies.
- Interactions between chamomile and cyclosporine (a drug used to prevent rejection of organ transplants) and warfarin (a blood thinner) have been reported, and there are theoretical reasons to suspect that chamomile might interact with other drugs as well. Talk to your healthcare provider before taking chamomile if you are taking any type of medicine.
- Little is known about whether it is safe to use chamomile during pregnancy or while breastfeeding.

KEEP IN MIND

- Take charge of your health—talk with your healthcare providers about any complementary health approaches you use. Together, you can make shared, well-informed decisions.

Section 22.9 | **Are Nutritional Supplements Useful Adjuncts?**

"Are Nutritional Supplements Useful Adjuncts?" © 2020 Omnigraphics. Reviewed August 2020.

Any person can be affected by anxiety, causing them to experience extreme fear, worry, panic, or unease. Though there are many treatment options for anxiety disorder—including therapy, medication, or a combination of both, research has suggested that many nutritional supplements, such as magnesium, omega-3 fatty acids, inositol, lysine, zinc, etc., can help alleviate the symptoms of anxiety.

VITAMINS AND SUPPLEMENTS THAT HELP COMBAT ANXIETY

Here are some evidence-based nutritional supplements that have proven to help relieve the symptoms of anxiety.

Magnesium

This is a mineral that helps improve the functioning of almost every system in our body. Some studies suggest that magnesium can ease the symptoms associated with anxiety.

- A systematic review compared the results of 18 studies and found that magnesium can help reduce anxiety in those who are more at risk of developing it.
- Another study suggests that women affected by anxiety due to premenstrual syndrome showed improvement after taking magnesium supplements.

It has arrived from these studies that since magnesium helps improve the brain functions, it reduces the level of anxiety in a person. Some type of magnesium considered best for anxiety are:

- Magnesium glycinate
- Magnesium oxide
- Magnesium citrate
- Magnesium chloride
- Magnesium sulfate (Epsom salt)
- Magnesium lactate

Not everyone is required to take magnesium supplements; instead, they can choose foods that are high in this nutrient. Some of these foods include:

- Whole wheat
- Spinach
- Quinoa
- Nuts such as almonds and cashews
- Dark chocolate
- Black beans

However, beware of taking a high dosage of magnesium as it can cause diarrhea. It is advised to start with a dosage as low as 100 milligrams (mg) and never exceed 350 mg per day without the doctor's consent.

Omega-3 Fatty Acids

This nutrient plays a significant role in strengthening the brain health; hence, it can help improve anxiety.

- A systematic review and meta-analysis saw results that suggest a regular intake of omega-3 supplements such as fish oil, helps people with anxiety.

Majority of such studies were done comparing omega-3 supplements to a placebo. However, it is too soon to recommend a high dosage of omega-3 supplements to treat anxiety since some further clinical trials and research have to be done.

Since our body cannot produce these fats, we must gain them from our diet. Foods such as fish and flaxseed are rich in omega-3 fats.

Inositol

This nutrient seems to have a positive effect on those affected by panic disorder. However, the impact that this has on people with other anxiety-related conditions such as obsessive-compulsive disorder (OCD) is still under research. An evidence that supports the theory that it helps those with panic disorder is:

- 21 patients with panic disorder were randomly given 6 gm of inositol or placebo twice a day for four weeks, which was later switched to other substances. It was noticed that the frequency and intensity of the attacks were significantly reduced in the group that had inositol.

Though there are mild side effects that have been reported by individuals who have taken inositol, no serious adverse effects have been observed. The same level of dosage prescribed for panic disorder is considered to be safe.

Zinc

There are extensive data available showing that mood disorders are linked with a significant reduction in the level of essential nutrients in the body, including zinc. Hence, the natural conclusion is that proper supply of this nutrient can help improve anxiety in a person.

Zinc helps maintain a healthy nervous system, especially the vagus nerve that connects the brain to the rest of the body. This is the nerve that transmits the "calm" messages to the body. A healthy nervous system contributes to a reduction in the level of anxiety. When a person is worried, the body uses all the zinc stored, attempting to keep the body relaxed. Some foods that are high in source of zinc are:

- Oysters
- Red meat
- Lentils
- Kidney beans
- Eggs
- Pumpkin seeds
- Sunflower seeds
- Cashew
- Mushroom
- Spinach

Though these nutritional supplements may help with the anxiety symptoms; however, it is always best to consult your physician about the frequency and amount to be taken before taking such supplements.

References

1. Berry, Jennifer. "Top 10 Evidence Based Supplements for Anxiety," Medical News Today, July 22, 2019.
2. "The Efficacy and Safety of Nutrient Supplements in the Treatment of Mental Disorders: A Meta-Review of Meta-Analyses of Randomized Controlled Trials," National Center for Biotechnology Information (NCBI), U.S. National Library of Medicine, September 9, 2019.
3. Walle, Gavin. "7 Best Vitamins and Supplements to Combat Stress," Healthline Media, November 18, 2019.
4. "Herbal and Dietary Supplements for Treatment of Anxiety Disorders," Healthline Media, August 15, 2007.
5. Ferguson, Sian. "Magnesium for Anxiety: Is It Effective?" Healthline Media, March 20, 2019.
6. "Omega-3s for Anxiety?" Harvard Health Publishing, Harvard Medical School, January 2019.
7. Lake, James. "Inositol: A Promising Treatment for Panic Disorder," *Psychology Today*, October 10, 2018.
8. "Could a Zinc Deficiency Contribute to Anxiety & Low Mood?" BePure, January 26, 2020.

Section 22.10 | Art and Play Therapy: Addressing Anxiety in Children

"Art and Play Therapy: Addressing Anxiety in Children," © 2020 Omnigraphics. Reviewed August 2020.

Anxiety often has a significant impact on children since they are not always capable of expressing their troubles. This is because they do not possess the verbal skills to describe their feelings, or they are often unsure of how they feel. Art and play therapy can be useful in such cases, providing children with a format that allows them to communicate their feelings effectively. It can help bridge the gap between the therapist and child by removing the language barrier and any other deterrents that prevent the child from sharing. It also helps children who feel afraid to share their suppressed feelings by giving them a safe emotional distance and protective environment away from their anxiety issues.

ART THERAPY FOR TREATING ANXIETY IN CHILDREN

This form of therapy is considered a very effective treatment for children with anxiety disorders due to its nonthreatening approach based on creative expression. It is necessary for anxious children to have a sense of safety in their surroundings to create artwork. There are several ways to let the child feel comfortable during an art therapy session, such as establishing that the child's work of art is not to be judged as "good" or "bad." When determining the progress of art therapy, the aesthetic quality and the technique used in the artwork are not considered as essential factors.

Benefits

Art therapy can help children learn more about their anxiety and ways of coping with it. The following are some of the benefits of art therapy for children.

- **Nonverbal communication.** It enables nonverbal communication of thoughts, emotions, and unconscious symbols and images that enables the therapist to gain a deeper understanding of the child's inner thinking.
- **Safe form of expression.** Art reflects the child's internal conflict and helps them externally represent and physically record their experience and emotions. Art therapy can be considered a safe place to contain the feelings of the child while processing.
- **Creates self-awareness.** Art therapy encourages the child to be creative, self-discover, problem-solve, and resolve conflicts.

PLAY THERAPY FOR TREATING ANXIETY IN CHILDREN

Play therapy is an expressive therapy similar to art therapy that provides a comprehensive view of the current level of a child's functionality. Making use of creative interventions in play therapy recognizes the relationship between body movement and storytelling. When acting out a narrative or portraying a character, the child is immersed in the story, imitating how they play in school or at home. Playing games, such as "tea party" or "house" lets children socialize and represent roles that can assist in forming their sense of identity in the future.

Benefits

Play therapy uses the attributes of a child's playtime to expand the therapeutic values of dealing with their anxiety. It can help children develop positive qualities that can help tackle anxiety disorders.

- **Enhanced social skills.** It enables a child to adapt to new surroundings and improves their social skills by helping them relax.
- **Assess and control situations.** It can help a child measure and evaluate the level of worry caused by their anxiety and maintain calm during stressful situations.
- **Cognitive restructuring.** This can be done using specially designed activities to identify and change or overcome a child's anxious thoughts or feelings.
- **Self-soothing.** This involves teaching a child how to regain their sense of calm using relaxation techniques such as taking deep breaths or through kinesthetic and tactile touch.
- **Distraction.** This can help the child divert their thinking away from anxious thoughts.
- **Positive reinforcement.** Constantly praising the child or rewarding them will help them experience a sense of mastery and increased self-esteem since anxious children often feel they are inadequate.

References

1. Wonders, Lynn. "Play Therapy Interventions for Anxiety," Wonders Counselling, July 30, 2018.
2. Messmer, Kaitilin. "Art and Play Therapy for Children with Anxiety," Digital Commons, October 15, 2010.
3. Eddins, Rachel. "Therapy for My Child: What are Art and Play Therapy?" Eddins Counselling Group, November 21, 2016.

Chapter 23 | **Support Groups**

If you have, or believe you may have, mental-health problem, it can be helpful to talk about these issues with others. It can be scary to reach out for help, but it is often the first step to helping you heal, grow, and recover.

Having a good support system and engaging with trustworthy people are key elements to successfully talking about your own mental health.

BUILD YOUR SUPPORT SYSTEM

Find someone—such as a parent, family member, teacher, faith leader, healthcare provider or other trusted individual, who:

- Gives good advice when you want and ask for it; assists you in taking action that will help
- Likes, respects, and trusts you and who you like, respect, and trust, too
- Allows you the space to change, grow, make decisions, and even make mistakes
- Listens to you and shares with you, both the good and bad times
- Respects your need for confidentiality so you can tell her or him anything

This chapter contains text excerpted from the following sources: Text in this chapter begins with excerpts from "For People with Mental Health Problems," MentalHealth.gov, U.S. Department of Health and Human Services (HHS), July 11, 2017; Text under the heading "School-Based Supports" is excerpted from "School-Based Supports," Youth.gov, October 8, 2017.

- Lets you freely express your feelings and emotions without judging, teasing, or criticizing
- Works with you to figure out what to do the next time a difficult situation comes up
- Has your best interest in mind

FIND A PEER GROUP

Find a group of people with mental-health problems similar to yours. Peer support relationships can positively affect individual recovery because:

- People who have common life experiences have a unique ability to help each other based on a shared history and a deep understanding that may go beyond what exists in other relationships
- People offer their experiences, strengths, and hopes to peers, which allows for natural evolution of personal growth, wellness promotion, and recovery
- Peers can be very supportive since they have "been there" and serve as living examples that individuals can and do recover from mental-health problems
- Peers also serve as advocates and support others who may experience discrimination and prejudice

You may want to start or join a self-help or peer support group. National organizations across the country have peer support networks and peer advocates.

SCHOOL-BASED SUPPORTS
Schools Are a Natural Setting to Support Mental Health

School-based mental health is becoming a vital part of student support systems. According to the most recent data in 2005, over one-third of school districts used school or district staff to provide mental-health services, and over one-fourth used outside agencies to provide mental-health services in the schools. The President's Now Is the Time plan to improve access to mental healthcare in our schools and communities emphasizes the urgency to "make sure students and young adults get treatment for mental-health issues" through early identification, referral for treatment, training for school teachers in early detection and response to mental illness, assistance for schools to address pervasive violence, and training for additional mental-health professionals to provide mental-health services in schools. Federal agencies, such as the President's New Freedom Commission on Mental Health, the U.S. Department of Health and Human Services (HHS), and the Institute of Medicine are also calling on schools to enhance early identification methods to assess and connect students with mental health.

Mentally healthy students are more likely to go to school ready to learn, actively engage in school activities, have supportive and caring connections with adults and young people, use appropriate problem-solving skills, have nonaggressive behaviors, and add to positive school culture. Although many students are mentally healthy, the Center for Mental Health in Schools estimates that between 12 and 22 percent of school-aged children and youth have a diagnosable mental-health disorder. Because children and youth spend the majority of their time in school, schools play an increasingly critical role in supporting these students and providing a safe, nonstigmatizing, and supportive natural environment in which children, youth, and families have access to prevention, early intervention, and treatment through school-based mental-health programs. A study by the U.S. Department of Health and Human Services Office of Adolescent Health indicated that adolescents are more comfortable accessing healthcare services through school-based clinics and like the idea of accessing a range of health and social services in a single location. Further, schools provide a natural setting in which students can receive needed supports and services and where families are comfortable and trusting in accessing these supports and services.

Implementing School-Based Mental-Health Services

The ways school districts implement school-based mental-health services vary. They may hire school-based therapists or social workers. They can provide access to prevention programming, early identification of mental-health challenges, and treatment options.

They can also partner with community mental-health organizations and agencies to develop an integrated, comprehensive program of support and services to do the following:

- Develop evidence-based programs to provide positive school climate and promote student skills in dealing with bullying and conflicts, solving problems, developing healthy peer relationships, engaging in activities to prevent suicide and substance use, and so on.
- Develop early intervention services for students in need of additional supports such as skill groups to deal with grief, anger, anxiety, sadness, and so on.
- Develop treatment programs and services that address the various mental-health needs of students.
- Develop student and family supports and resources.
- Develop a school culture in which teachers and other student support staff are trained to recognize the early warning signs of mental-health issues with students.
- Develop a referral process to ensure that all students have equal access to services and supports.

Further, early identification and referral resources may reflect a school climate that is comfortable talking about and addressing emotional health, which again may reduce the stigma often associated with receiving mental-health treatment.

Benefits of School-Based Mental-Health Services

Studies have shown the value of developing comprehensive school mental-health programs in helping students achieve academically and have access to experiences that build social skills, leadership, self-awareness, and caring connections to adults in their school and community. Schools that also choose to collaborate with community partners have found that they can enhance the academic success of individual students. These partnerships have found to significantly improve schoolwide truancy and discipline rates, increase the rates of high school graduation, and help create a positive school environment in which a student can learn and be successful in school and in the community.

Chapter 24 | Integrating Behavioral Health Services into Primary Care

Integrated Care combines primary healthcare and mental healthcare in one setting. There are many ways to integrate care, and they may go by different names, including "collaborative care" or "health homes." This is an important model of care because:

- Primary care settings, such as a doctor's office, provide about half of all mental healthcare for common psychiatric disorders.
- Adults with serious mental illnesses and substance-use disorders (SUD) also have higher rates of chronic physical illnesses and die earlier than the general population.
- People with common physical-health conditions also have higher rates of mental-health issues.

Providing Integrated Care helps patients and their providers. It blends the expertise of mental health, substance use, and primary care clinicians, with feedback from patients and their caregivers. This creates a team-based approach where mental healthcare and

This chapter contains text excerpted from the following sources: Text in this chapter begins with excerpts from "Integrated Care," National Institute of Mental Health (NIMH), February 2017; Text beginning with the heading "What Is Behavioral Health Integration?" is excerpted from "Adding Better Mental Healthcare to Primary Care," National Institute of Mental Health (NIMH), December 30, 2016. Reviewed August 2020.

general medical care are offered in the same setting. Coordinating primary care and mental healthcare in this way can help address the physical-health problems of people with serious mental illnesses.

WHY IS IT IMPORTANT?

Addressing the whole person and her or his physical and behavioral health is essential for positive health outcomes and cost-effective care. Many people may not have access to mental healthcare or may prefer to visit their primary healthcare provider. Although most primary care providers can treat mental disorders, particularly through medication, that may not be enough for some patients. Historically, it has been difficult for a primary care provider to offer effective, high-quality mental healthcare when working alone. Combining mental-health services/expertise with primary care can reduce costs, increase the quality of care, and, ultimately, save lives.

Addressing Physical and Behavioral Health

Untreated or undertreated mental illnesses have serious conse-quences. People with severe mental illness often die 13 to 30 years earlier than the general population from medical conditions that could have been treated by a primary care provider.

Treating Children

Most children with mental-health conditions are treated in a primary care setting instead of a specialized mental-health setting. About half of all mental-health disorders begin by 14 years of age. Accurate diagnoses and quality care are vital in a primary care setting.

Treating Adults

Adults are also more likely to be seen in a primary care setting than within a mental-health system. Primary care providers deliver half of the mental healthcare for common conditions such as anx-iety, attention deficit hyperactivity disorder (ADHD), depression, behavioral problems, and substance use. Yet, people with mental illnesses who are treated in a primary care setting are less likely to receive effective behavioral healthcare. For example, 75 percent of adult patients with depression see primary care providers, but only half are accurately diagnosed. When a referral is made to a mental-health provider, only about half of patients follow through with making an appointment. As a result, many behavioral-health problems go undetected, undertreated, and/or untreated.

HOW DOES IT WORK?

Integrated Care meets all of a patient's health needs in one setting. It can be delivered in multiple ways depending on who is providing the care, what type of care is being provided, where the care is taking place, and how services are being coordinated. Integration can take place in behavioral health, primary care, specialty clinics, and home health settings.

There are different levels of services integration. The Substance Abuse and Mental Health Service Administration (SAMHSA) designed a framework to help healthcare providers plan and support an integrated system. That framework has three main categories:

- Coordinated Care, which concentrates on communication
- Co-located Care, which focuses on physical proximity
- Integrated Care, which emphasizes practice change

Within each category, there are varying degrees of collaboration between care providers. These levels range from minimal to full integration. Minimal integration is when medical and mental healthcare providers work in separate facilities, have separate systems, and rarely communicate. Full integration involves a single health system's medical and mental healthcare providers working simultaneously to treat a patient's behavioral and medical needs with shared medical record access.

The following are examples of Integrated Care programs:

Collaborative Care

A team-based collaborative care program adds two new types of services to usual primary care: behavioral-healthcare management and consultations with a mental-health specialist.

The behavioral-healthcare manager becomes part of the patient's treatment team and helps the primary care provider evaluate the patient's mental health. If the patient receives a diagnosis of a mental-health disorder, and wants treatment, the care manager, primary care provider, and patient work together to develop a treatment plan. This plan may include medication, psychotherapy, or other appropriate options.

Later, the care manager reaches out to see if the patient likes the plan, is following the plan, and if the plan is working or if changes are needed. The care manager and the primary care provider also regularly review the patient's status and care plan with a mental-health specialist, like a psychiatrist or psychiatric nurse, to be sure the patient is getting the best treatment options and improving.

Patient-Centered Medical Home

Another Integrated Care model is the patient-centered medical home (PCMH). PCMH involves coordinating a patient's overall healthcare needs at any age. Patients play active roles in their healthcare. Providers coordinate all aspects of preventive, acute, and chronic needs of patients using the best available evidence and appropriate technology.

As a result of the Affordable Care Act (ACA), health homes were established for individuals on Medicaid with chronic conditions including mental health and SUDs, asthma, diabetes, heart disease, and obesity. Health homes are team-based with a whole-person approach with specific emphasis on integrating behavioral health and primary care. Health homes provide comprehensive-care management, coordination, and follow-up. They also offer patient and family support, referrals to community and support services, and health promotion.

Hub-Based Systems

Found mostly in the child mental-health world, hub-based systems modeled on the Massachusetts Child Psychiatry Access Project (MCPAP) provide primary care providers with immediate telephone consultations with a child psychiatrist. Case management and face-to-face evaluations are also available for complicated cases.

Four Quadrant Model

The Four Quadrant Model is a way to measure an organization's level of integration.

The Four Quadrant Clinical Integration Model describes integration levels in terms of primary care and behavioral-healthcare complexity and risk. The location, types of providers, and services vary depending on the complexity of patients' conditions.

For instance, individuals with mild-to-moderate physical and/or behavioral-health issues may be best cared for in a primary care setting with integrated behavioral-health providers. For patients with complex general medical conditions as well as mild-to-moderate behavioral-health disorders, a medical specialty setting with integrated behavioral-health providers may be appropriate. Those with severe behavioral problems as well as medical conditions may receive the most comprehensive care in a specialty behavioral-health center with integrated general medical providers, or a health home.

Pediatric versus Adult Integrated Care

Pediatric Integrated Care differs from adult Integrated Care in three main ways:

There is an increased sensitivity to how children are developing, both mentally and emotionally.
- Families play an important role.
- Treatment emphasizes coping and adjustment techniques in addition to standard care.

The general principles of Integrated Care apply to adults as well as children and adolescents, but work with developing youth and their families is often different from the work with adults with complex medical illness. In addition, ongoing evaluation for intellectual disability and developmental delays will be emphasized in pediatric evaluations.

WHAT IS BEHAVIORAL HEALTH INTEGRATION?

Many people visit a primary healthcare provider (such as a doctor, nurse practitioner, or physician assistant) to treat physical diseases and injuries. However, it is also common for patients to see a primary care provider because of behavioral-health issues including mental illnesses such as depression, anxiety, or problems with alcohol use. The primary care provider can treat mental disorders, particularly through medication, but that may not be enough. Historically, it has been difficult for a primary care provider alone to offer effective, high-quality behavioral healthcare.

Integrating a "Collaborative Care" approach is one proven way primary care providers can enhance the quality and effectiveness of their behavioral health treatment. A team-based Collaborative Care program adds two new types of services to usual primary care: behavioral healthcare management and consultations with a mental-health specialist.

WHAT IS NEW?

The Centers for Medicare and Medicaid Services (CMS) has adopted a new coverage policy for Medicare. On January 1, 2017, CMS began paying primary care clinicians separately for Collaborative Care services that they provide to patients who are being treated for a mental- or behavioral-health condition. There are other ways a primary care provider can integrate mental-health services, but this policy change emphasizes Collaborative Care, including services from a primary care provider, a behavioral healthcare manager, and consultations with mental-health specialists.

WHY IS THIS IMPORTANT?

Medicare's new payment policy for behavioral health integration will have an immediate effect on those healthcare providers who are already offering mental healthcare to their clients. However, this new policy may have a much wider impact. It may increase the number of healthcare providers who offer behavioral healthcare to their Medicare clients and improve access to high-quality care for patients across the country. Currently, it is believed that only about 10 percent of patients with depression receive appropriate mental healthcare when visiting their primary healthcare provider. Medicare's new payment program may also encourage private insurance companies to offer similar payment options for integrating behavioral healthcare with primary care visits.

Part 4 | Psychiatric Comorbidities in Anxiety Disorder

Chapter 25 | Comorbidities of Anxiety Disorders

Comorbidity is a state of having more than one medical condition at the same time. A. R. Feinstein, a famous American doctor and epidemiologist, first created the term "comorbidity" in 1970s. He further demonstrated through an example of rheumatic fever, how multiple other diseases are comorbid (coexisting) with it. The term is frequently used in both medicine and psychology.

COMORBIDITIES OF GENERALIZED ANXIETY DISORDER

Generalized anxiety disorder (GAD) is the most common anxiety disorder and has the highest comorbidity rate than any other anxiety disorder. Major depressive disorder (MDD), substance-use disorder (SUD), and bipolar disorder (BD) are the most common GAD comorbidities.

Generalized Anxiety Disorder and Bipolar Disorder

Categorized by a severe shift in mood, bipolar disorder was previously known as "manic depression" due to the extreme highs and lows in a person's mood. Bipolar disorder affects a person's capacity to execute everyday tasks, such as school or work and make it difficult to maintain relationships. Studies have shown that 51 percent of patients with BD also have another anxiety disorder, which worsens their condition. When experiencing a high, the person can be over ecstatic, and at their low, then can be suicidal for no reason. Research reveals that the number of suicide attempts in patients with current and lifetime GAD comorbidity is higher in BD patients alone. As a result, the patients experience a lower quality of life, lower chance of recovery, and increased risk of substance abuse and suicidal tendencies.

Generalized Anxiety Disorder and Major Depressive Disorder

A person suffering from GAD is in a continual state of worry when there might be nothing to worry about. GAD develops slowly, starting in the early teen or young adult years. Daily life such as schoolwork, family, job, finance, or fear of the future may keep a person in a state of perpetual angst that interferes with their daily activities. MDD is also known as "clinical depression" or "depression." It is a mood disorder that causes noticeable problems in a person's day-to-day activities and relationships with others. The person may also have trouble making decisions and feel angry or irritated for no reason. MDD also affects a person's ability to concentrate. It makes it difficult for an individual to cheer up and makes them feel hopeless for a prolonged period. A person diagnosed with GAD and MDD is at an increased risk for suicidality and severe functional impairment. Even with increased medication, this syndrome is difficult to treat and has a more extended remission period.

Generalized Anxiety Disorder and Substance-Use disorder

Research has identified a link between patients with GAD and substance-abuse tendencies. Initially, those suffering from anxiety are unaware that they might have an anxiety disorder, and so they try things like drugs, alcohol, and self-medication to ease themselves. After using these substances for a while, the individual's body builds a tolerance for these substances and they need to increase their usage to achieve the same results. This leads to their dependence on substance use leading to SUD. There is a three-way correlative pattern that can be observed between these two disorders:

- Anxiety leading to substance use
- Substance use leading to anxiety
- Genetic risk that is central to both the disorders (GAD and SUD)

Often people may consume a pint of beer or a glass of wine to calm their nerves, but drinking alcohol in large quantities over a long period of time is said to increase anxiety. Because of its ability to cause anxiety, alcohol can have a serious effect on a person's health especially if they suffer from GAD. Similarly, the use of marijuana provides a temporary relief after a stressful day or situation. Once the "high" effect is gone, feelings of anxiety often return and the individual may begin to use marijuana on a regular basis to feel calm.

COMORBIDITIES OF SOCIAL ANXIETY DISORDER

People with a social anxiety disorder (SAD) have an increased chance of being predisposed to another disorder, making treatment a bit complex. Other disorders comorbid with SAD are as follows:

- **Depression.** People with SAD are likely to develop depression later in life because their condition makes them live in a state of constant fear of being judged or rejected. If a person is only treated for depression and not for SAD, the treatment will not be fully effective and may cause a relapse. That is why it is important to share all your symptoms with your healthcare provider.
- **Panic disorder (PD).** Someone diagnosed with SAD can also have PD. There may be some differences in the panic triggers and symptoms experienced by someone with SAD and PD. However, the treatment for both may or may not be the same. People with PD may avoid meeting new people or trying new things in life out of fear or worry that triggers a panic attack.
- **Avoidant personality disorder (APD).** People with APD may experience similar symptoms as someone with SAD, and because of this overlap, APD is considered comorbid with SAD. However, the symptoms of APD may be more severe and broader. While those with SAD feel that others will humiliate or judge them, people with APD think that others cannot be trusted with their motives, which marks a significant difference between SAD and APD.

197

- **Schizophrenia.** Little has been researched about SAD and schizophrenia as a comorbidity, but there is some evidence linking the two together. Like all other disorders, people with both SAD and schizophrenia have a lower quality of life.
- **Eating disorders.** Some people with SAD may also develop eating disorders like binge eating disorder, bulimia nervosa, and anorexia nervosa. Some people might fear to eat in public, but the motivation behind someone suffering from SAD is different.

COMORBIDITY OF AGORAPHOBIA WITH PANIC DISORDER AND SOCIAL ANXIETY DISORDER

Most people think agoraphobia is the fear of leaving one's house, whereas it is the fear of being stuck in places or situations where escape will be difficult if they had a panic attack. This leads them to be housebound and such individuals prefer leaving the house with a trusted companion rather than by themselves. People with agoraphobia may fear being in crowded places, riding public transport, being in an elevator, or a movie theatre.

However, SAD also includes fear of public places but only in situations where they feel others will judge them. A person with SAD will not be afraid to commute in the bus or ride an elevator.

References

1. Smith, Yolanda. "Generalized Anxiety Disorder Comorbidities," News Medical Life Sciences, February 2019.
2. Cuncic, Arlin. "7 Disorders Related to Social Anxiety Disorder," Very Well Mind, February 2020.
3. Cameron, Oliver G. "Understanding Comorbid Depression and Anxiety," Psychiatric Times, December 2007.
4. Cuncic, Arlin. "The Relationship Between Agoraphobia and Social Anxiety," Very Well Mind, July 2019.

5. "Everything You Need to Know About Bipolar Disorder," Healthline, January 2018.
6. "Agoraphobia," Mayo Clinic, November 2017.
7. Ellis, Mary Ellen. "Why Co-Occurring Generalized Anxiety and Depression Need Comprehensive Treatment," Bridges to Recovery, February 2019.
8. Christiansen, Thomas. "Generalized Anxiety Disorder and Substance Abuse," The Recovery Village, January 2020.

Chapter 26 | The Connection between ADHD and Anxiety

DISORDERS ASSOCIATED WITH ADHD[1]

Attention deficit hyperactivity disorder (ADHD) often occurs with other disorders. Many children with ADHD have other disorders as well as ADHD such as behavior or conduct problems, learning disorders, anxiety, and depression.

The combination of ADHD with other disorders often presents extra challenges for children, parents, educators, and healthcare providers. Therefore, it is important for healthcare providers to screen every child with ADHD for other disorders and problems. This chapter provides an overview of the more common conditions and concerns that can occur with ADHD. Talk with your healthcare provider if you have concerns about your child's symptoms.

WHAT IS ADHD?[2]

Attention deficit hyperactivity disorder is one of the most common neurodevelopmental disorders of childhood. It is usually first diagnosed in childhood and often lasts into adulthood. Children with ADHD may have trouble paying attention, controlling impulsive

This chapter includes text excerpted from documents published by two public domain sources. Text under the headings marked 1 are excerpted from "Other Concerns and Conditions with ADHD," Centers for Disease Control and Prevention (CDC), August 27, 2019; Text under the headings marked 2 are excerpted from "What Is ADHD?" Centers for Disease Control and Prevention (CDC), April 8, 2020.

behaviors (may act without thinking about what the result will be), or be overly active.

SIGNS AND SYMPTOMS OF ATTENTION DEFICIT HYPERACTIVITY DISORDER[2]

It is normal for children to have trouble focusing and behaving at one time or another. However, children with ADHD do not just grow out of these behaviors. The symptoms continue, can be severe, and can cause difficulty at school, at home, or with friends.

A child with ADHD might:

- Daydream a lot
- Forget or lose things a lot
- Squirm or fidget
- Talk too much
- Make careless mistakes or take unnecessary risks
- Have a hard time resisting temptation
- Have trouble taking turns
- Have difficulty getting along with others

CAUSES OF ATTENTION DEFICIT HYPERACTIVITY DISORDER[2]

Scientists are studying cause(s) and risk factors in an effort to find better ways to manage and reduce the chances of a person having ADHD. The cause(s) and risk factors for ADHD are unknown, but current research shows that genetics plays an important role.

In addition to genetics, scientists are studying other possible causes and risk factors including:

- Brain injury
- Exposure to environmental (e.g., lead) during pregnancy or at a young age
- Alcohol and tobacco use during pregnancy
- Premature delivery
- Low birth weight

Research does not support the popularly held views that ADHD is caused by eating too much sugar, watching too much television, parenting, or social and environmental factors such as poverty or family chaos. Of course, many things, including these, might make symptoms worse, especially in certain people. But, the evidence is not strong enough to conclude that they are the main causes of ADHD.

TYPES OF ATTENTION DEFICIT HYPERACTIVITY DISORDER[2]

There are three different types of ADHD, depending on which types of symptoms are strongest in the individual.

- **Predominantly inattentive presentation.** It is hard for the individual to organize or finish a task, to pay attention to details, or to follow instructions or conversations. The person is easily distracted or forgets details of daily routines.
- **Predominantly hyperactive-impulsive presentation.** The person fidgets and talks a lot. It is hard to sit still for long (e.g., for a meal or while doing homework). Smaller children may run, jump, or climb constantly. The individual feels restless and has trouble with impulsivity. Someone who is impulsive may interrupt others a lot, grab things from people, or speak at inappropriate times. It is hard for the person to wait for their turn or listen to directions. A person with impulsiveness may have more accidents and injuries than others.
- **Combined presentation.** Symptoms of the above two types are equally present in the person.

Because symptoms can change over time, the presentation may change over time as well.

ANXIETY AND DEPRESSION[1]
Anxiety

Many children have fears and worries. However, when a child experiences so many fears and worries that they interfere with school, home, or play activities, it is an anxiety disorder. Children with ADHD are more likely than those without to develop an anxiety disorder.

Examples of anxiety disorders include:

- **Separation anxiety**—being very afraid when they are away from family
- **Social anxiety**—being very afraid of school and other places where they may meet people
- **General anxiety**—being very worried about the future and about bad things happening to them

Depression

Occasionally being sad or feeling hopeless is a part of every child's life. When children feel persistent sadness and hopelessness, it can cause problems. Children with ADHD are more likely than children without ADHD to develop childhood depression. Children may be more likely to feel hopeless and sad when they cannot control their ADHD symptoms and the symptoms interfere with doing well at school or getting along with family and friends.

Examples of behaviors often seen when children are depressed include:

- Feeling sad or hopeless a lot of the time
- Not wanting to do things that are fun
- Having a hard time focusing
- Feeling worthless or useless

Children with ADHD often have a hard time focusing on things that are not very interesting to them. Depression can make it hard to focus on things that are normally fun. Changes in eating and sleeping habits can also be a sign of depression. For children with ADHD who take medication, changes in eating and sleeping can also be side effects from the medication rather than signs of depression. Talk with your healthcare provider if you have concerns. Extreme depression can lead to thoughts of suicide.

Treatment for Anxiety and Depression

The first step to treatment is to talk with a healthcare provider to get an evaluation. Some signs of depression, such as having a hard time focusing, are also signs of ADHD, so it is important to get a careful evaluation to see if a child has both conditions. A mental-health professional can develop a therapy plan that works best for the child and family. Early treatment is important, and can include child therapy, family therapy, or a combination of both. The school can also be included in therapy programs. For very young children, involving parents in treatment is very important. Cognitive-behavioral therapy (CBT) is one form of therapy that is used to treat anxiety or depression, particularly in older children. It helps the child change negative thoughts into more positive, effective ways of thinking. Consultation with a health provider can help determine if medication should also be part of the treatment.

Chapter 27 | **Bipolar Disorder**

WHAT IS BIPOLAR DISORDER?

Bipolar disorder is a chronic or episodic (which means occurring occasionally and at irregular intervals) mental disorder. It can cause unusual, often extreme and fluctuating changes in mood, energy, activity, and concentration or focus. The bipolar disorder sometimes is called "manic-depressive disorder" or "manic depression," which are older terms.

Everyone goes through normal ups and downs, but bipolar disorder is different. The range of mood changes can be extreme. In manic episodes, someone might feel very happy, irritable, or "up," and there is a marked increase in activity level. In depressive episodes, someone might feel sad, indifferent, or hopeless, in combination with a very low activity level. Some people have hypomanic episodes, which are like manic episodes, but less severe and troublesome.

Most of the time, the bipolar disorder develops or starts during late adolescence (teen years) or early adulthood. Occasionally, bipolar symptoms can appear in children. Although the symptoms come and go, bipolar disorder usually requires lifetime treatment and does not go away on its own. Bipolar disorder can be an important factor in suicide, job loss, and family discord, but proper treatment leads to better outcomes.

This chapter includes text excerpted from "Bipolar Disorder," National Institute of Mental Health (NIMH), October 2018.

WHAT ARE THE SYMPTOMS OF BIPOLAR DISORDER?

The symptoms of bipolar disorder can vary. An individual with bipolar disorder may have manic episodes, depressive episodes, or "mixed" episodes. A mixed episode has both manic and depressive symptoms. These mood episodes cause symptoms that last a week or two or sometimes longer. During an episode, the symptoms last every day for most of the day. Mood episodes are intense. The feelings are intense and happen along with changes in behavior, energy levels, or activity levels that are noticeable to others.

Symptoms of a Manic Episode

- Feeling very up, high, elated, or extremely irritable or touchy
- Feeling jumpy or wired, more active than usual
- Racing thoughts
- Decreased need for sleep
- Talking fast about a lot of different things ("flight of ideas")
- Excessive appetite for food, drinking, sex, or other pleasurable activities
- Thinking you can do a lot of things at once without getting tired
- Feeling like you are unusually important, talented, or powerful

Symptoms of a Depressive Episode

- Feeling very down or sad, or anxious
- Feeling slowed down or restless
- Trouble concentrating or making decisions
- Trouble falling asleep, waking up too early, or sleeping too much
- Talking very slowly, feeling like you have nothing to say, or forgetting a lot
- Lack of interest in almost all activities
- Unable to do even simple things
- Feeling hopeless or worthless, or thinking about death or suicide

Some people with bipolar disorder may have milder symptoms than others with the disorder. For example, hypomanic episodes may make the individual feel very good and be very productive; they may not feel like anything is wrong. However, family and friends may notice the mood swings and changes in activity levels as behavior that is different from usual, and severe depression may follow mild hypomanic episodes.

HOW IS BIPOLAR DISORDER TREATED?

Treatment helps many people, even those with the most severe forms of bipolar disorder. Doctors treat bipolar disorder with medications, psychotherapy, or a combination of treatments.

Medications

Certain medications can help control the symptoms of bipolar disorder. Some people may need to try several different medications and work with their doctor before finding the ones that work best. The most common types of medications that doctors prescribe include mood stabilizers and atypical antipsychotics. Mood stabilizers such as lithium can help prevent mood episodes or reduce their severity when they occur. Lithium also decreases the risk for suicide. Additional medications that target sleep or anxiety are sometimes added to mood stabilizers as part of a treatment plan.

Talk with your doctor or a pharmacist to understand the risks and benefits of each medication. Report any concerns about side effects to your doctor right away. Avoid stopping medication without talking to your doctor first.

Psychotherapy

Psychotherapy (sometimes called "talk therapy") is a term for a variety of treatment techniques that aim to help a person identify and change troubling emotions, thoughts, and behaviors. Psychotherapy can offer support, education, skills, and strategies to people with bipolar disorder and their families. Psychotherapy often is used in combination with medications; some types of psychotherapy (e.g., interpersonal, social rhythm therapy) can be an effective treatment for bipolar disorder when used with medications.

Other Treatments

Some people may find other treatments helpful in managing their bipolar symptoms, including:

- Electroconvulsive therapy is a brain stimulation procedure that can help people get relief from severe symptoms of bipolar disorder. This type of therapy is usually considered only if a patient's illness has not improved after other treatments (such as medication or psychotherapy) are tried, or in cases where rapid response is needed, as in the case of suicide risk and catatonia (a state of unresponsiveness), for example.
- Regular vigorous exercise such as jogging, swimming, or bicycling, helps with depression and anxiety, promotes better sleep, and is healthy for your heart and brain. Check with your doctor before you start a new exercise regimen.
- Keeping a life chart, which records daily mood symptoms, treatments, sleep patterns, and life events, can help people and their doctors track and treat bipolar disorder.

Not much research has been conducted on herbal or natural supplements and how they may affect bipolar disorder. Talk to your doctor before taking any supplement. Certain medications and supplements taken together can cause serious side effects or life-threatening drug reactions.

Finding Treatment

The National Institute of Mental Health (NIMH) is a federal research agency and cannot provide medical advice or referrals to practitioners. However, there are tools and resources available that may help you find a provider or treatment.

You can also:
- Call your doctor. Your doctor can be the first step in getting help.
- Call the Substance Abuse and Mental Health Services Administration (SAMHSA) Treatment Referral Helpline at 800-662-HELP (800-662-4357) for general information on mental health and to find local treatment services.
- Visit the SAMHSA website (findtreatment.samhsa. gov), which has a Behavioral Health Treatment Services Locator that can search for treatment information by address, city, or ZIP code.
- Seek immediate help from a doctor or the nearest hospital emergency room, or call 911, if you or someone you know is in crisis or considering suicide.

Coping with Bipolar Disorder

Living with bipolar disorder can be challenging, but there are ways to help make it easier for yourself, a friend, or a loved one.
- Get treatment and stick with it—recovery takes time and it is not easy. But, treatment is the best way to start feeling better.
- Keep medical and therapy appointments, and talk with the provider about treatment options.
- Take all medicines as directed.
- Structure activities: keep a routine for eating and sleeping, and make sure to get enough sleep and exercise.
- Learn to recognize your mood swings.
- Ask for help when trying to stick with your treatment.
- Be patient; improvement takes time. Social support helps.

Remember, bipolar disorder is a lifelong illness, but long-term, ongoing treatment can help control symptoms and enable you to live a healthy life.

Chapter 28 | **Borderline Personality Disorder**

WHAT IS BORDERLINE PERSONALITY DISORDER?

Borderline personality disorder (BPD) is an illness marked by an ongoing pattern of varying moods, self-image, and behavior. These symptoms often result in impulsive actions and problems in relationships with other people. A person with BPD may experience episodes of anger, depression, and anxiety that may last from a few hours to days. Recognizable symptoms typically show up during adolescence (teenage years) or early adulthood, but early symptoms of the illness can occur during childhood.

WHAT ARE THE SIGNS AND SYMPTOMS?

People with BPD may experience mood swings and may display uncertainty about how they see themselves and their role in the world. As a result, their interests and values can change quickly. People with BPD also tend to view things in extremes, such as all good or all bad. Their opinions of other people can also change quickly. An individual who is seen as a friend one day may be considered an enemy or traitor the next. These shifting feelings can lead to intense and unstable relationships.

This chapter includes text excerpted from "Borderline Personality Disorder," National Institute of Mental Health (NIMH), December 7, 2017.

Other signs or symptoms may include:

- Efforts to avoid real or imagined abandonment such as rapidly initiating intimate (physical or emotional) relationships or cutting off communication with someone in anticipation of being abandoned
- A pattern of intense and unstable relationships with family, friends, and loved ones, often swinging from extreme closeness and love (idealization) to extreme dislike or anger (devaluation)
- Distorted and unstable self-image or sense of self
- Impulsive and often dangerous behaviors such as spending sprees, unsafe sex, substance abuse, reckless driving, and binge eating. **Note:** If these behaviors occur primarily during times of elevated mood or energy, they may be indicative of a mood disorder, rather than borderline personality disorder.
- Self-harming behavior, such as cutting
- Recurring thoughts of suicidal behaviors or threats
- Intense and highly changeable moods, with each episode lasting from a few hours to a few days
- Chronic feelings of emptiness
- Inappropriate, intense anger or problems controlling anger
- Difficulty trusting, which is sometimes accompanied by irrational fear of other people's intentions
- Feelings of dissociation, such as feeling cut off from oneself, observing oneself from outside one's body, or feelings of unreality

Not everyone with BPD experiences every symptom. Some individuals experience only a few symptoms, while others have many. Symptoms can be triggered by seemingly ordinary events; for example, people with BPD may become angry and distressed over minor separations—due to business trips or changes in plans—from people to whom they feel close. The severity and frequency of symptoms and how long they last will vary depending on the individual and their particular illness.

WHAT CAUSES BORDERLINE PERSONALITY DISORDER

Scientists are not sure what causes BPD, but research suggests that genetic, environmental, and social factors play a role.

- **Family history.** People who have a close family member (such as a parent or sibling) with the disorder may be at a higher risk of developing BPD or traits of BPD (such as impulsiveness and aggression).
- **Brain factors.** Studies show that people with BPD can have structural and functional changes in the brain especially in the areas that control impulses and emotional regulation. But, it is not clear whether these changes were risk factors for the disorder, or caused by the disorder.
- **Environmental, cultural, and social factors.** Many people with BPD report experiencing traumatic life events such as abuse, abandonment, or adversity during childhood. Others may have been exposed to unstable, invalidating relationships, and hostile conflicts.

Although these factors may increase a person's risk, it does not mean that the person will develop BPD. Likewise, there may be people without these risk factors who will develop BPD in their lifetime.

HOW DO YOU KNOW IF YOU HAVE BORDERLINE PERSONALITY DISORDER?

A licensed mental-health professional—such as a psychiatrist, psychologist, or clinical social worker—experienced in diagnosing and treating mental disorders can diagnose BPD, based on a thorough interview and a discussion about symptoms. A careful and thorough medical exam can also help rule out other possible causes of symptoms.

The mental-health professional may ask about symptoms and personal and family medical histories, including any history of mental illness. This information can help determine the best treatment.

What Other Illnesses Often Co-occur with Borderline Personality Disorder?

Borderline personality disorder often occurs with other mental illnesses. These co-occurring disorders can make it harder to diagnose and treat BPD, especially if symptoms of other illnesses overlap with the symptoms of BPD. For example, a person with BPD may be more likely to also experience symptoms of major depression, bipolar disorder, anxiety disorders, substance abuse, or eating disorders.

HOW IS BORDERLINE PERSONALITY DISORDER TREATED?

Borderline personality disorder has historically been viewed as difficult to treat. But with newer, evidence-based treatment (EBT), many people with BPD experience fewer and less severe symptoms, improved functioning, and an improved quality of life (QOL). It is important for patients with BPD to receive evidence-based, specialized treatment from an appropriately-trained mental-health professional. Other types of treatment, or treatment provided by a provider who is not appropriately trained, may not benefit the patient.

Many factors affect the length of time it takes for symptoms to improve once treatment begins, so it is important for people with BPD and their loved ones to be patient and to receive appropriate support during treatment.

It Is Important to Seek—and Stick with—Treatment

The National Institute of Mental Health (NIMH)-funded studies indicate that BPD patients who do not receive adequate treatment are more likely to develop other chronic medical or mental illnesses and are less likely to make healthy lifestyle choices. BPD is also associated with a significantly higher rate of self-harm and suicidal behavior than the general population.

The treatments described below are just some of the options that may be available to a person with borderline personality disorder.

Psychotherapy

Psychotherapy is the first-line treatment for people with BPD. It can be provided one-on-one between the therapist and the patient or in a group setting. Therapist-led group sessions may help teach people with BPD how to interact with others and how to express themselves effectively. It is important that people in therapy get along with and trust their therapist. The very nature of BPD can make it difficult for people with this disorder to maintain a comfortable and trusting bond with their therapist.

Two examples of psychotherapies used to treat BPD include dialectical behavior therapy (DBT) and cognitive-behavioral therapy (CBT).

Dialectical behavior therapy, which was developed for individuals with BPD, uses concepts of mindfulness and acceptance or being aware of and attentive to the current situation and emotional state. DBT also teaches skills to control intense emotions, reduce self-destructive behaviors, and improve relationships.

Cognitive-behavioral therapy can help people with BPD identify and change core beliefs and behaviors that underlie inaccurate perceptions of themselves and others and problems interacting with others. CBT may help reduce a range of mood and anxiety symptoms and reduce the number of suicidal or self-harming behaviors.

Medications

Medications are not typically used as the primary treatment for BPD as the benefits are unclear. However, in some cases, a psychiatrist may recommend medications to treat specific symptoms such as mood swings, depression, or other mental disorders that may occur with BPD. Treatment with medications may require care from more than one medical professional.

Certain medications can cause different side effects in different people. Individuals should talk to her or his provider about what to expect from a particular medication.

Other Elements of Care

Some people with BPD experience severe symptoms and require intensive, often inpatient, care. Other people may need outpatient treatments but never need hospitalization or emergency care.

Therapy for Caregivers and Family Members

Families of people with BPD may also benefit from therapy. Having a relative with the disorder can be stressful, and family members may unintentionally act in ways that worsen their relative's symptoms.

Some BPD therapies include family members in treatment sessions. These sessions help families develop skills to better understand and support a relative with BPD. Other therapies focus on the needs of family members to help them understand the obstacles and strategies for caring for someone with BPD. Although more research is needed to determine the effectiveness of family therapy in BPD, studies on other mental disorders suggest that including family members can help in a person's treatment.

Chapter 29 | **Depression**

Anxiety disorders commonly occur along with other mental illnesses, including alcohol abuse, which may mask anxiety symptoms or make them worse. In some cases, these other illnesses need to be treated in order to have a full response to treatment directed at the target anxiety disorder. Patients with underlying anxiety disorders frequently display somatic complaints that are the subject of visits to the primary care office.

WHAT IS DEPRESSION?

Depression is more than just feeling down or having a bad day. When a sad mood lasts for a long time and interferes with normal, everyday functioning, you may be depressed. Symptoms of depression include:
- Feeling sad or anxious often or all the time
- Not wanting to do activities that used to be fun
- Feeling irritable' easily frustrated' or restless
- Having trouble falling asleep or staying asleep
- Waking up too early or sleeping too much
- Eating more or less than usual or having no appetite
- Experiencing aches, pains, headaches, or stomach problems that do not improve with treatment
- Having trouble concentrating, remembering details, or making decisions
- Feeling tired' even after sleeping well

This chapter contains text excerpted from the following sources: Text in this chapter begins with excerpts from "Depression and Anxiety Management Search—Volume 2," Mental Illness Research, Education, and Clinical Centers (MIRECC), U.S. Department of Veterans Affairs (VA), January 31, 2013. Reviewed August 2020; Text beginning with the heading "What Causes Depression" is excerpted from "Mental Health Conditions: Depression and Anxiety," Centers for Disease Control and Prevention (CDC), March 23, 2020.

- Feeling guilty, worthless, or helpless
- Thinking about suicide or hurting yourself

The following information is not intended to provide a medical diagnosis of major depression and cannot take the place of seeing a mental-health professional. If you think you are depressed' talk with your doctor or a mental-health professional immediately. This is especially important if your symptoms are getting worse or affecting your daily activities.

WHAT CAUSES DEPRESSION

The exact cause of depression is unknown. It may be caused by a combination of genetic, biological, environmental, and psychological factors. Everyone is different' but the following factors may increase a person's chances of becoming depressed:

- Having blood relatives who have had depression
- Experiencing traumatic or stressful events, such as physical or sexual abuse, the death of a loved one, or financial problems
- Going through a major life change' even if it was planned
- Having a medical problem, such as cancer, stroke, or chronic pain
- Taking certain medications. Talk to your doctor if you have questions about whether your medications might be making you feel depressed.
- Using alcohol or drugs

WHO GETS DEPRESSION

In general' about 1 out of every 6 adults will have depression at some time in their life. Depression affects about 16 million American adults every year. Anyone can get depressed, and depression can happen at any age and in any type of person.

Many people who experience depression also have other mental-health conditions. Anxiety disorders often go hand in hand with depression. People who have anxiety disorders struggle with intense and uncontrollable feelings of anxiety, fear, worry, and/or panic. These feelings can interfere with daily activities and may last for a long time.

WHAT ARE THE TREATMENTS FOR DEPRESSION?

Many helpful treatments for depression are available. Treatment for depression can help reduce symptoms and shorten how long the depression lasts. Treatment can include getting therapy and/or taking medications. Your doctor or a qualified mental-health professional can help you determine what treatment is best for you.

Therapy

Many people benefit from psychotherapy—also called "therapy" or "counseling." Most therapy lasts for a short time and focuses on thoughts' feelings' and issues that are happening in your life now. In some cases, understanding your past can help' but finding ways to address what is happening in your life now can help you cope and prepare you for challenges in the future. With therapy, you will work with your therapist to learn skills to help you cope with life, change behaviors that are causing problems' and find solutions. Do not feel shy or embarrassed about talking openly and honestly about your feelings and concerns This is an important part of getting better. Some common goals of therapy include:

- Getting healthier
- Quitting smoking and stopping drug and alcohol use
- Overcoming fears or insecurities
- Coping with stress
- Making sense of past painful events
- Identifying things that worsen your depression
- Having better relationships with family and friends
- Understanding why something bothers you and creating a plan to deal with it

Medication

Many people with depression find that taking prescribed medications called "antidepressants" can help improve their mood and coping skills. Talk to your doctor about whether they are right for

you. If your doctor writes you a prescription for an antidepressant'
ask exactly how you should take the medication. If you are already
using nicotine replacement therapy or another medication to help
you quit smoking, be sure to let your doctor know. Several antidepressant medications are available' so you and your doctor have
options to choose from. Sometimes it takes several tries to find the
best medication and the right dose for you, so be patient. Also, be
aware of the following important information:

- When taking these medications' it is important to
  follow the instructions on how much to take. Some
  people start to feel better a few days after starting the
  medication' but it can take up to four weeks to feel the
  most benefit. Antidepressants work well and are safe
  for most people' but it is still important to talk with
  your doctor if you have side effects. Side effects usually
  do not get in the way of daily life' and they often go
  away as your body adjusts to the medication.

- Do not stop taking an antidepressant without first
  talking to your doctor. Stopping your medicine
  suddenly can cause symptoms or worsen depression.
  Work with your doctor to safely adjust how much you
  take.

- Some antidepressants may cause risks during
  pregnancy. Talk with your doctor if you are pregnant
  or might be pregnant, or if you are planning to become
  pregnant.

- Antidepressants cannot solve all of your problems. If
  you notice that your mood is getting worse or if you
  have thoughts about hurting yourself' it is important to
  call your doctor right away.

Chapter 30 | Eating Disorders

Eating disorders have a high degree of comorbidity with other psychiatric disorders, as well as with some medical disorders. In anorexia nervosa, affective disorders are most common, followed by anxiety disorders with obsessive-compulsive disorder (OCD) most prevalent. Among patients suffering from bulimia nervosa, high rates of affective disorder and anxiety disorders have been reported, as well as personality disorders and substance abuse. Binge Eating disorder is associated with a higher degree of psychiatric comorbidity than is found in people who are obese who do not binge eat. Also, a "failure to thrive" syndrome, characterized by malnutrition, depression, and physical illness has been described in geriatric populations. Despite their high degree of comorbidity, eating disorders are distinct disorders; they do not transmute into other illnesses.

AN OVERVIEW OF EATING DISORDERS

There is a commonly held misconception that eating disorders are a lifestyle choice. Eating disorders are actually serious and often fatal illnesses that are associated with severe disturbances in people's eating behaviors and related thoughts and emotions. Preoccupation with food, body weight, and shape may also signal

This chapter contains text excerpted from the following sources: Text in this chapter begins with excerpts from "Mental-Health Research in Eating Disorders," National Institutes of Health (NIH), July 12, 1996. Reviewed August 2020; Text beginning with the heading "An Overview of Eating Disorders" is excerpted from "Eating Disorders," National Institute of Mental Health (NIMH), February 2016. Reviewed August 2020; Text under the heading "Comorbidity with Other Mental Disorders in Adults" is excerpted from "Eating Disorders," National Institute of Mental Health (NIMH), November 2017.

an eating disorder. Common eating disorders include anorexia nervosa, bulimia nervosa, and binge eating disorder.

SIGNS AND SYMPTOMS OF EATING DISORDERS
Anorexia Nervosa

People with anorexia nervosa may see themselves as overweight, even when they are dangerously underweight. People with anorexia nervosa typically weigh themselves repeatedly, severely restrict the amount of food they eat, often exercise excessively, and/or may force themselves to vomit or use laxatives to lose weight. Anorexia nervosa has the highest mortality rate of any mental disorder. While many people with this disorder die from complications associated with starvation, others die of suicide.

Symptoms include:
- Extremely restricted eating
- Extreme thinness (emaciation)
- A relentless pursuit of thinness and unwillingness to maintain a normal or healthy weight
- Intense fear of gaining weight
- Distorted body image, a self-esteem that is heavily influenced by perceptions of body weight and shape, or a denial of the seriousness of low body weight

Other symptoms may develop over time, including:
- Thinning of the bones (osteopenia or osteoporosis)
- Mild anemia and muscle wasting and weakness
- Brittle hair and nails
- Dry and yellowish skin
- Growth of fine hair all over the body (lanugo)
- Severe constipation
- Low blood pressure, slowed breathing and pulse
- Damage to the structure and function of the heart
- Brain damage
- Multiorgan failure
- Drop in internal body temperature, causing a person to feel cold all the time
- Lethargy, sluggishness, or feeling tired all the time
- Infertility

Bulimia Nervosa

People with bulimia nervosa have recurrent and frequent episodes of eating unusually large amounts of food and feeling a lack of control over these episodes. This binge eating is followed by behavior that compensates for the overeating such as forced vomiting, excessive use of laxatives or diuretics, fasting, excessive exercise, or a combination of these behaviors. People with bulimia nervosa may be slightly underweight, normal weight, or over overweight.

Symptoms include:
- Chronically inflamed and sore throat
- Swollen salivary glands in the neck and jaw area
- Worn tooth enamel and increasingly sensitive and decaying teeth as a result of exposure to stomach acid
- Acid reflux disorder and other gastrointestinal problems
- Intestinal distress and irritation from laxative abuse
- Severe dehydration from purging of fluids
- Electrolyte imbalance (too low or too high levels of sodium, calcium, potassium, and other minerals) which can lead to stroke or heart attack

Binge Eating Disorder

People with binge eating disorder lose control over her or his eating. Unlike bulimia nervosa, periods of binge eating are not followed by purging, excessive exercise, or fasting. As a result, people with Binge Eating disorder often are overweight or obese. Binge Eating disorder is the most common eating disorder in the United States.

Symptoms include:
- Eating unusually large amounts of food in a specific amount of time, such as a two-hour period
- Eating even when you are full or not hungry
- Eating fast during binge episodes
- Eating until you are uncomfortably full
- Eating alone or in secret to avoid embarrassment
- Feeling distressed, ashamed, or guilty about your eating
- Frequently dieting, possibly without weight loss

RISK FACTORS OF EATING DISORDERS

Eating disorders can affect people of all ages, racial/ethnic backgrounds, body weights, and genders. Eating disorders frequently appear during the teen years or young adulthood but may also develop during childhood or later in life. These disorders affect both genders, although rates among women are higher than among men. Like women who have eating disorders, men also have a distorted sense of body image.

Researchers are finding that eating disorders are caused by a complex interaction of genetic, biological, behavioral, psychological, and social factors. Researchers are using the latest technology and science to better understand eating disorders.

One approach involves the study of human genes. Eating disorders run in families. Researchers are working to identify deoxyribonucleic acid (DNA) variations that are linked to the increased risk of developing eating disorders.

Brain imaging studies are also providing a better understanding of eating disorders. For example, researchers have found differences in patterns of brain activity in women with eating disorders in comparison with healthy women. This kind of research can help guide the development of new means of diagnosis and treatment of eating disorders.

TREATMENTS AND THERAPIES OF EATING DISORDERS

It is important to seek treatment early for eating disorders. People with eating disorders are at higher risk for suicide and medical complications. People with eating disorders can often have other mental disorders (such as depression or anxiety) or problems with substance use. Complete recovery is possible.

Treatment plans are tailored to individual needs and may include one or more of the following:

- Individual, group, and/or family psychotherapy
- Medical care and monitoring
- Nutritional counseling
- Medications

Psychotherapies

Psychotherapies such as a family-based therapy called the "Maudsley approach," where parents of adolescents with anorexia nervosa assume responsibility for feeding their child, appear to be very effective in helping people gain weight and improve eating habits and moods.

To reduce or eliminate Binge Eating and purging behaviors, people may undergo cognitive-behavioral therapy (CBT), which is another type of psychotherapy that helps a person learn how to identify distorted or unhelpful thinking patterns and recognize and change inaccurate beliefs.

Medications

Evidence also suggests that medications such as antidepressants, antipsychotics, or mood stabilizers may also be helpful for treating eating disorders and other co-occurring illnesses, such as anxiety or depression.

COMORBIDITY WITH OTHER MENTAL DISORDERS IN ADULTS

Based on diagnostic interview data from the National Comorbidity Survey Replication (NCS-R), table 30.1. shows the lifetime comorbidity of eating disorders with core mental disorders in the fourth edition of the *Diagnostic and Statistical Manual of Mental Disorders* (DSM-IV).

- More than half (56.2%) of respondents with anorexia nervosa, (94.5%) with bulimia nervosa, and (78.9%) with BED met criteria for at least one of the core DSM-IV disorders assessed in the NCS-R.
- All three eating disorders had the highest comorbidity with any anxiety disorder.

Table 30.1. Lifetime Comorbidity with Other Mental Disorders in Adults

	Anorexia Nervosa (%)	Bulimia Nervosa (%)	Binge Eating Disorder (%)
Any Anxiety Disorder	47.9	80.6	65.1
Any Mood Disorder	42.1	70.7	46.4
Any Impulse Control Disorder	30.8	63.8	43.3
Any Substance-Use Disorder	27	36.8	23.3
Any Disorder	56.2	94.5	78.9

Chapter 31 | **Illness Anxiety Disorder**

WHAT IS ILLNESS ANXIETY DISORDER?

Illness anxiety disorder is a condition in which a person is preoccupied with having or acquiring a serious disease. The person misinterprets normal body sensations, or minor symptoms, as indications of major illness, even though a thorough medical examination fails to reveal any serious disease. People with a high risk of acquiring a medical condition, in particular, become consumed with worry and often assume various normal bodily sensations are symptoms of the disease. This leads to anxiety that is more severe than the physical symptoms themselves and causes distress that can affect a person's daily life. The disorder occurs in early adulthood and may be seen in both men and women.

The condition that was previously known as "hypochondriasis" has been reclassified in the *Diagnostic and Statistical Manual of Mental Disorders, 5th Edition* (DSM-5) of the American Psychiatric Association (APA) under the following two disorders:

- **Illness anxiety disorder**, which manifests with mild or no physical symptoms
- **Somatic symptom disorder**, which manifests with multiple, sometimes major, physical symptoms

Note that illness anxiety disorder and somatic symptom disorder are different conditions in that physical symptoms are usually

"Illness Anxiety Disorder," © 2018 Omnigraphics. Reviewed August 2020.

not seen in illness anxiety disorder, while they are present, and significantly so, in somatic symptom disorder.

WHAT ARE THE SYMPTOMS OF ILLNESS ANXIETY DISORDER?

People with illness anxiety disorder worry about getting a serious disease and so are preoccupied with related thoughts, causing distress that can impair work, family, and social life. Physical symptoms may or may not be present, although they are usually relatively mild. Patients are generally more concerned about the implications of the symptoms rather than the symptoms themselves.

They get easily alarmed about their health, and negative medical test results fail to provide any reassurance. Patients may frequently consult many healthcare professionals for reassurance, or they might avoid medical care altogether for fear of being diagnosed with a serious illness. Some patients examine themselves obsessively for new symptoms by looking in the mirror or checking their skin for lesions. They think that any new symptom or sensation is a sign of serious illness.

Illness anxiety disorder is chronic, sometimes fluctuating in some people while remaining steady in others. Some patients are able to understand their fears are unreasonable and unfounded, and many of these individuals tend to recover.

WHAT CAUSES ILLNESS ANXIETY DISORDER

The exact causes of illness anxiety disorder are not known, but the following factors likely play a role:

- **Lack of education.** A poor understanding of disease and what body sensations actually mean could contribute to misinterpretation of symptoms.
- **Learned behavior.** A parent or other family member with excessive anxiety about health issues could promote similar behavior in relatives.
- **Past experiences.** Serious illnesses in childhood could make individuals susceptible to frightening thoughts about physical sensations.

WHAT ARE THE RISK FACTORS OF ILLNESS ANXIETY DISORDER?

The following are some of the risk factors of illness anxiety disorder:

- A period of life spent with high stress
- The threat of illness that existed but did not become serious
- A history of child abuse
- A history of illness in childhood or a parent with serious illness
- The personality trait of being a worrier
- The tendency to check the Internet obsessively, searching for illnesses

HOW IS ILLNESS ANXIETY DISORDER DIAGNOSED?

As part of diagnosis, a healthcare professional will conduct a complete physical examination and routine medical tests to find out if the patient has any condition that requires treatment. In the absence of any such condition, the patient will likely be referred to a mental healthcare professional for further diagnosis.

A psychiatrist, psychologist, or other mental-health specialist will conduct a psychological evaluation and elicit information on symptoms, family history, fears and concerns, stress factors, relationship problems, and other issues in the patient's life. The diagnosis will then be made based on criteria defined in the DSM-5. Some factors considered for diagnosis include preoccupation with symptoms lasting for at least six months, no somatic symptoms or minimal somatic symptoms, fear of acquiring a serious illness, and the absence of any other mental-health condition.

HOW IS ILLNESS ANXIETY DISORDER TREATED?

The goal of treatment is to help the patient lead a normal life. Psychotherapy, especially cognitive-behavioral therapy (CBT), is used to deal with emotional aspects of the disorder. The patient is taught to recognize symptoms, deal with them, and lead an active life even if symptoms persist. Sometimes antidepressants or other medications are prescribed to help relieve symptoms.

WHAT IS THE PROGNOSIS FOR ILLNESS ANXIETY DISORDER?

Illness anxiety disorder could become a chronic condition unless the psychological factors causing the disorder are treated, so continuing to work with trained professionals is the key to a successful outcome. Stress management and relaxation techniques may help reduce anxiety, and staying physically active can improve mood and reduce stress. In addition, the use of alcohol and recreational drugs can aggravate symptoms and increase anxiety, so these should be avoided.

References

1. "Illness Anxiety Disorder," Mayo Foundation for Medical Education and Research (MFMER), July 2, 2015.
2. Dimsdale, Joel E., MD. "Illness Anxiety Disorder," Merck & Co., August 2016.
3. Berger, Fred K., MD. "Illness Anxiety Disorder," A.D.A.M., Inc., July 29, 2016.

Chapter 32 | **Obsessive-Compulsive Disorder and Anxiety**

Obsessive-compulsive disorder (OCD) is a common, chronic (long-lasting) disorder in which a person has uncontrollable, re-occurring thoughts (obsessions) and behaviors (compulsions) that she or he feels the urge to repeat over and over in response to the obsession.

While everyone sometimes feels the need to double check things, people with OCD have uncontrollable thoughts that cause them anxiety, urging them to check things repeatedly or perform routines and rituals for at least 1 hour per day. Performing the routines or rituals may bring brief but temporary relief from the anxiety. However, left untreated, these thoughts and rituals cause the person great distress and get in the way of work, school, and personal relationships.

WHAT ARE THE SIGNS AND SYMPTOMS OF OBSESSIVE-COMPULSIVE DISORDER?

People with OCD may have obsessions, compulsions, or both. Some people with OCD also have a tic disorder. Motor tics are sudden, brief, repetitive movements such as eye blinking, facial grimacing,

This chapter contains text excerpted from the following sources: Text in this chapter begins with excerpts from "Obsessive-Compulsive Disorder: When Unwanted Thoughts or Irresistible Actions Take Over," National Institute of Mental Health (NIMH), 2016. Reviewed August 2020; Text beginning with the heading Obsessive-Compulsive Disorder in Children" is excerpted from "Obsessive-Compulsive Disorder in Children," Centers for Disease Control and Prevention (CDC), March 30, 2020.

shoulder shrugging, or head or shoulder jerking. Common vocal tics include repetitive throat-clearing, sniffing, or grunting sounds.

Obsessions may include:
- Fear of germs or contamination
- Fear of losing or misplacing something
- Worries about harm coming towards oneself or others
- Unwanted and taboo thoughts involving sex, religion, or others
- Having things symmetrical or in perfect order

Compulsions may include:
- Excessively cleaning or washing a body part
- Keeping or hoarding unnecessary objects
- Ordering or arranging items in a particular, precise way
- Repeatedly checking on things, such as making sure that the door is locked or the oven is off
- Repeatedly counting items
- Constantly seeking re-assurance

WHAT CAUSES OBSESSIVE-COMPULSIVE DISORDER

Obsessive-compulsive disorder may have a genetic component. It sometimes runs in families, but no one knows for sure why some family members have it while others do not. OCD usually begins in adolescence or young adulthood, and tends to appear at a younger age in boys than in girls. Researchers have found that several parts of the brain, as well as biological processes, play a key role in obsessive thoughts and compulsive behavior, as well as the fear and anxiety related to them. Researchers also know that people who have suffered physical or sexual trauma are at an increased risk for OCD.

OBSESSIVE-COMPULSIVE DISORDER IN CHILDREN

Many children occasionally have thoughts that bother them, and they might feel like they have to do something about those thoughts, even if their actions do not actually make sense. For example, they might worry about having bad luck if they do not wear a favorite piece of clothing. For some children, the thoughts and the urges to perform certain actions persist, even if they try to ignore them or make them go away. Children may have an OCD when unwanted thoughts, and the behaviors they feel they must do because of the thoughts, happen frequently, take up a lot of time (more than an hour a day), interfere with their activities, or make them very upset. The thoughts are called "obsessions." The behaviors are called "compulsions."

TREATMENTS FOR OBSESSIVE-COMPULSIVE DISORDER

The first step to treatment is to talk with a healthcare provider to arrange an evaluation. A comprehensive evaluation by a mental-health professional will determine if the anxiety or distress involves memories of a traumatic event that actually happened, or if the fears are based on other thoughts or beliefs. The mental-health professional should also determine whether someone with OCD has a current or past tic disorder. Anxiety or depression and disruptive behaviors may also occur with OCD.

Treatments can include behavior therapy and medication. Behavior therapy, specifically cognitive-behavioral therapy, helps the child change negative thoughts into more positive, effective ways of thinking, leading to more effective behavior. Behavior therapy for OCD can involve gradually exposing children to their fears in a safe setting; this helps them learn that bad things do not really occur when they do not do the behavior, which eventually decreases their anxiety. Behavior therapy alone can be effective, but some children are treated with a combination of behavior therapy and medication. Families and schools can help children manage stress by being part of the therapy process and learning how to respond supportively without accidentally making obsessions or compulsions more likely to happen again.

Chapter 33 | **Posttraumatic Stress Disorder**

Posttraumatic stress disorder (PTSD) is a disorder that develops in some people who have experienced a shocking, scary, or dangerous event.

It is natural to feel afraid during and after a traumatic situation. Fear triggers many split-second changes in the body to help defend against danger or to avoid it. This "fight-or-flight" response is a typical reaction meant to protect a person from harm. Nearly everyone will experience a range of reactions after trauma, yet most people recover from initial symptoms naturally. Those who continue to experience problems may be diagnosed with PTSD. People who have PTSD may feel stressed or frightened, even when they are not in danger.

SIGNS AND SYMPTOMS OF POSTTRAUMATIC STRESS DISORDER

While most but not all traumatized people experience short-term symptoms, the majority do not develop ongoing (chronic) PTSD. Not everyone with PTSD has been through a dangerous event. Some experiences, such as the sudden, unexpected death of a loved one, can also cause PTSD. Symptoms usually begin early, within three months of the traumatic incident, but sometimes they begin years afterward. Symptoms must last more than a month and be severe enough to interfere with relationships or work to be considered PTSD. The course of the illness varies. Some people recover

This chapter contains text excerpted from the following sources: Text in this chapter begins with excerpts from "Post-Traumatic Stress Disorder," National Institute of Mental Health (NIMH), May 2019; Text beginning with the heading "Active Coping" is excerpted from "Coping with Traumatic Stress Reactions," National Center for Posttraumatic Stress Disorder (NCPTSD), U.S. Department of Veterans Affairs (VA), January 13, 2020.

within six months, while others have symptoms that last much longer. In some people, the condition becomes chronic.

A doctor who has experience helping people with mental illnesses, such as a psychiatrist or psychologist, can diagnose PTSD.

To be diagnosed with PTSD, an adult must have all of the following for at least a month:
- At least one re-experiencing symptom
- At least one avoidance symptom
- At least two arousal and reactivity symptoms
- At least two cognition and mood symptoms

Re-experiencing symptoms include:
- Flashbacks—reliving the trauma over and over, including physical symptoms such as a racing heart or sweating
- Bad dreams
- Frightening thoughts

Re-experiencing symptoms may cause problems in a person's everyday routine. The symptoms can start from the person's own thoughts and feelings. Words, objects, or situations that are reminders of the event can also trigger re-experiencing symptoms.

Avoidance symptoms include:
- Staying away from places, events, or objects that are reminders of the traumatic experience
- Avoiding thoughts or feelings related to the traumatic event

Things that remind a person of the traumatic event can trigger avoidance symptoms. These symptoms may cause a person to change her or his personal routine. For example, after a bad car accident, a person who usually drives may avoid driving or riding in a car.

Arousal and reactivity symptoms include:
- Being easily startled
- Feeling tense or "on edge"
- Having difficulty sleeping
- Having angry outbursts

Arousal symptoms are usually constant, instead of being triggered by things that remind one of the traumatic events. These symptoms can make the person feel stressed and angry. They may make it hard to do daily tasks, such as sleeping, eating, or concentrating.

Cognition and mood symptoms include:

- Trouble remembering the key features of the traumatic event
- Negative thoughts about oneself or the world
- Distorted feelings such as guilt or blame
- Loss of interest in enjoyable activities

Cognition and mood symptoms can begin or worsen after the traumatic event, but are not due to injury or substance use. These symptoms can make the person feel alienated or detached from friends or family members.

It is natural to have some of these symptoms for a few weeks after a dangerous event. When the symptoms last more than a month, seriously affect one's ability to function, and are not due to substance use, medical illness, or anything except the event itself, they might be PTSD. Some people with PTSD do not show any symptoms for weeks or months. PTSD is often accompanied by depression, substance abuse, or one or more of the other anxiety disorders.

Do Children React Differently than Adults?

Children and teens can have extreme reactions to trauma, but some of their symptoms may not be the same as adults. Symptoms sometimes seen in very young children (less than 6 years of age), these symptoms can include:

- Wetting the bed after having learned to use the toilet
- Forgetting how to or being unable to talk
- Acting out the scary event during playtime
- Being unusually clingy with a parent or other adult

Older children and teens are more likely to show symptoms similar to those seen in adults. They may also develop disruptive, disrespectful, or destructive behaviors. Older children and teens may feel guilty for not preventing injury or deaths. They may also have thoughts of revenge.

RISK FACTORS OF POSTTRAUMATIC STRESS DISORDER

Anyone can develop PTSD at any age. This includes war Veterans, children, and people who have been through a physical or sexual assault, abuse, accident, disaster, or other serious events. According to the National Center for PTSD, about 7 or 8 out of every 100 people will experience PTSD at some point in their lives. Women are more likely to develop PTSD than men, and genes may make some people more likely to develop PTSD than others.

Not everyone with PTSD has been through a dangerous event. Some people develop PTSD after a friend or family member experiences danger or harm. The sudden, unexpected death of a loved one can also lead to PTSD.

Why Do Some People Develop PTSD and Other People Do Not?

It is important to remember that not everyone who lives through a dangerous event develops PTSD. In fact, most people will not develop the disorder.

Many factors play a part in whether a person will develop PTSD. Some examples are listed below. Risk factors make a person more likely to develop PTSD. Other factors, called "resilience factors," can help reduce the risk of the disorder.

Some factors that increase the risk for PTSD include:

- Living through dangerous events and traumas
- Getting hurt
- Seeing another person hurt, or seeing a dead body
- Childhood trauma
- Feeling horror, helplessness, or extreme fear
- Having little or no social support after the event
- Dealing with extra stress after the event, such as loss of a loved one, pain and injury, or loss of a job or home
- Having a history of mental illness or substance abuse

Some factors that may promote recovery after trauma include:
- Seeking out support from other people, such as friends and family
- Finding a support group after a traumatic event
- Learning to feel good about one's own actions in the face of danger
- Having a positive coping strategy, or a way of getting through the bad event and learning from it
- Being able to act and respond effectively despite feeling fear
- Researchers are studying the importance of these and other risk and resilience factors, including genetics and neurobiology. With more research, someday it may be possible to predict who is likely to develop PTSD and to prevent it.

ACTIVE COPING
- Active coping means accepting the impact of trauma on your life and taking direct action to improve things.
- Active coping occurs even when there is no crisis. Active coping is a way of responding to everyday life. It is a habit that must be made stronger.

KNOW THAT RECOVERY IS A PROCESS
Following exposure to trauma most people experience stress reactions. Understand that recovering from the trauma is a process and takes time. Knowing this will help you feel more in control.
- Having an ongoing response to the trauma is normal.
- Recovery is an ongoing, daily process. It happens little by little. It is not a matter of being cured all of a sudden.
- Healing does not mean forgetting traumatic events. It does not mean you will have no pain or bad feelings when thinking about them.
- Healing may mean fewer symptoms and symptoms that bother you less.

- Healing means more confidence that you will be able to cope with your memories and symptoms. You will be better able to manage your feelings.

POSITIVE COPING ACTIONS

Certain actions can help to reduce your distressing symptoms and make things better. Plus, these actions can result in changes that last into the future. Here are some positive coping methods:

Learn about Trauma and PTSD

It is useful for trauma survivors to learn more about common reactions to trauma and about PTSD. Find out what is normal. Find out what the signs are that you may need assistance from others. When you learn that the symptoms of PTSD are common, you realize that you are not alone, weak, or crazy. It helps to know your problems are shared by hundreds of thousands of others. When you seek treatment and begin to understand your response to trauma, you will be better able to cope with the symptoms of PTSD.

Talk to Others for Support

When survivors talk about their problems with others, something helpful often results. It is important not to isolate yourself. Instead, make efforts to be with others. Of course, you must choose your support people with care. You must also ask them clearly for what you need. With support from others, you may feel less alone and more understood. You may also get concrete help with a problem you have.

Practice Relaxation Methods

Try some different ways to relax, including:
- Muscle relaxation exercises
- Breathing exercises
- Meditation
- Swimming, stretching, yoga
- Prayer

- Listening to quiet music
- Spending time in nature

While relaxation techniques can be helpful, in a few people they can sometimes increase distress at first. This can happen when you focus attention on disturbing physical sensations and you reduce contact with the outside world. Most often, continuing with relaxation in small amounts that you can handle will help reduce negative reactions. You may want to try mixing relaxation in with music, walking, or other activities.

Distract Yourself with Positive Activities

Pleasant recreational or work activities help distract a person from her or his memories and reactions. For example, art has been a way for many trauma survivors to express their feelings in a positive, creative way. Pleasant activities can improve your mood, limit the harm caused by PTSD, and help you rebuild your life.

Talking to Your Doctor or a Counselor about Trauma and PTSD

Part of taking care of yourself means using the helping resources around you. If efforts at coping do not seem to work, you may become fearful or depressed. If your PTSD symptoms do not begin to go away or get worse over time, it is important to reach out and call a counselor who can help turn things around. Your family doctor can also refer you to a specialist who can treat PTSD. Talk to your doctor about your trauma and your PTSD symptoms. That way, she or he can take care of your health better.

Many with PTSD have found treatment with medicines to be helpful for some symptoms. By taking medicines, some survivors of trauma are able to improve their sleep, anxiety, irritability, and anger. It can also reduce urges to drink or use drugs.

COPING WITH THE SYMPTOMS OF PTSD

Here are some direct ways to cope with these specific PTSD symptoms:

Unwanted distressing memories, images, or thoughts
- Remind yourself that they are just that, memories.
- Remind yourself that it is natural to have some memories of the trauma(s).
- Talk about them to someone you trust.
- Remember that, although reminders of trauma can feel overwhelming, they often lessen with time.

Sudden Feelings of Anxiety or Panic

Traumatic stress reactions often include feeling your heart pounding and feeling light-headed or spacey. This is usually caused by rapid breathing. If this happens, remember that:
- These reactions are not dangerous. If you had them while exercising, they most likely would not worry you.
- These feelings often come with scary thoughts that are not true. For example, you may think, "I'm going to die," "I'm having a heart attack," or "I will lose control." It is the scary thoughts that make these reactions so upsetting.
- Slowing down your breathing may help.
- The sensations will pass soon and then you can go on with what you were doing.

Each time you respond in these positive ways to your anxiety or panic, you will be working toward making it happen less often. Practice will make it easier to cope.

Feeling like the Trauma Is Happening Again (Flashbacks)
- Keep your eyes open. Look around you and notice where you are.
- Talk to yourself. Remind yourself where you are, what year you are in, and that you are safe. The trauma happened in the past, and you are in the present.
- Get up and move around. Have a drink of water and wash your hands.
- Call someone you trust and tell them what is happening.

- Remind yourself that this is a common response after trauma.
- Tell your counselor or doctor about the flashback(s).

Dreams and Nightmares Related to the Trauma

- If you wake up from a nightmare in a panic, remind yourself that you are reacting to a dream. Having the dream is why you are in a panic, not because there is real danger now.
- You may want to get up out of bed, regroup, and orient yourself to the here and now.
- Engage in a pleasant, calming activity. For example, listen to some soothing music.
- Talk to someone if possible.
- Talk to your doctor about your nightmares. Certain medicines can be helpful.

Irritability, Anger, and Rage

- Take a time out to cool off or think things over. Walk away from the situation.
- Get in the habit of exercise daily. Exercise reduces body tension and relieves stress.
- Remember that staying angry does not work. It actually increases your stress and can cause health problems.
- Talk to your counselor or doctor about your anger. Take classes on how to manage anger.
- If you blow up at family members or friends, find time as soon as you can to talk to them about it. Let them know how you feel and what you are doing to cope with your reactions.

Difficulty Concentrating or Staying Focused

- Slow down. Give yourself time to focus on what you need to learn or do.
- Write things down. Making "to-do" lists may be helpful.

- Break tasks down into small do-able chunks.
- Plan a realistic number of events or tasks for each day.
- You may be depressed. Many people who are depressed have trouble concentrating. Again, this is something you can discuss with your counselor, doctor, or someone close to you.

Trouble Feeling or Expressing Positive Emotions

- Remember that this is a common reaction to trauma. You are not doing this on purpose. You should not feel guilty for something you do not want to happen and cannot control.
- Make sure to keep taking part in activities that you enjoy or used to enjoy. Even if you do not think you will enjoy something, once you get into it, you may well start having feelings of pleasure.
- Take steps to let your loved ones know that you care. You can express your caring in little ways: write a card, leave a small gift, or phone someone and say hello.

Chapter 34 | Somatic Symptom Disorder

WHAT IS SOMATIC SYMPTOM DISORDER?

Somatic symptom disorder (formerly known as "hypochondria") is a condition in which an individual worry to an intense degree about having a physical illness that cannot be verified medically. The person becomes obsessed with the idea that physical symptoms such as pain, shortness of breath, or weakness, are due to serious disease, causing major distress to the point of disrupting daily life. The symptoms are not usually faked. They may or may not be related to a serious illness, but they do exist, and the individual truly believes she or he is sick. Somatic symptom disorder can occur at any age but is usually seen in early adulthood, affecting men and women equally. The disorder causes significant emotional and physical suffering, but its symptoms can be eased and the quality of life improved with proper treatment.

WHAT ARE THE SYMPTOMS OF SOMATIC SYMPTOM DISORDER?

Symptoms can vary considerably but typically may include:

- Pain
- Fatigue
- Weakness
- Shortness of breath
- Difficulty swallowing
- Nausea

"Somatic Symptom Disorders," © 2018 Omnigraphics. Reviewed August 2020.

- Dizziness
- Paralysis
- Vision problems
- Amnesia

The thoughts, feelings, and behaviors related to somatic symptom disorder can include one or more of the following:
- Significant worry that a potential illness exists
- Thoughts that physical symptoms are a sign of severe illness
- Frequently checking the body for symptoms
- Feeling that physical activity could worsen the condition
- Frequent healthcare visits that do not improve the condition
- Belief that doctors are failing to make an accurate diagnosis
- Consulting many doctors or "shopping around" for a doctor who agrees that the person has a serious illness
- Severe emotional and/or physical impairment unrelated to a medical condition
- Anxiety, nervousness, or depression that negatively affect everyday life

WHAT ARE THE RISK FACTORS FOR SOMATIC SYMPTOM DISORDER?

The following are some risk factors that are often associated with somatic symptom disorder:
- An existing medical condition or ongoing recovery from one
- Family history of disease or otherwise susceptible to a disease
- Genetic and biological factors that cause increased sensitivity to pain
- Anxiety or depression
- Recent stressful life events, such as violence or trauma
- History of childhood sexual abuse or other trauma

- Low socioeconomic status or education
- Learned behavior, such as receiving attention or other benefits from having an illness
- Problems in processing emotions, which causes pain to become the focus rather than the emotional problems

HOW IS SOMATIC SYMPTOM DISORDER DIAGNOSED?

It is difficult to diagnose somatic symptom disorder, in part because patients are convinced about the cause of their symptoms. Depending on the patient's symptoms, a healthcare professional will order tests and conduct a complete physical examination to rule out illness. In the absence of any detectable medical condition, the patient will likely be referred to a psychiatrist or other mental-health professional. The psychologist or psychiatrist will assess the person's attitude and behavior and will likely administer a personality assessment. The diagnosis of somatic symptom disorder is made on the basis of detailed criteria present in the *Diagnostic and Statistical Manual of Mental Disorders* (DSM-5), published by the American Psychiatric Association (APA).

HOW IS SOMATIC SYMPTOM DISORDER TREATED?

Somatic symptom disorder is treated with psychotherapy, usually cognitive-behavioral therapy, as well as with psychiatric medications.

Psychotherapy

The goal of psychotherapy is to help the patient live a productive life, even if the condition persists. It attempts to alter the thinking and behavior that lead to the symptoms. Treatment could be difficult because the patient firmly believes that symptoms are due to a physical illness and not the result of emotional or mental disturbances. Cognitive-behavioral therapy (CBT) helps patients reduce their preoccupation with symptoms and helps them cope with the ongoing condition. With stress-reduction techniques, patients are often able to improve their daily functioning at home, work, and in family life.

Medications

Psychiatric medications can help improve the condition of patients by reducing the symptoms associated with depression, anxiety, and pain. It may take several weeks for the medications to have the desired effect, and certain medicines may not be suitable in specific cases. The doctor may switch medications or alter combinations of drugs to improve their effectiveness.

HOW CAN SOMATIC SYMPTOM DISORDER BE PREVENTED?

Although not much information is available on the prevention of somatic symptom disorder, the following recommendations may be helpful:

- Seek professional help if you have anxiety or depression.
- Understand how stress affects the body, and learn to de-stress yourself by using stress-reduction techniques.
- If you think you might have somatic symptom disorder, seek medical help as early as possible to avoid worsening of symptoms and to ensure early recovery.
- Stick to the treatment plan.

References

1. "Somatic Symptom Disorder," American Psychiatric Association (APA), 2017.
2. "Somatic Symptom Disorder," Mayo Foundation for Medical Education and Research (MFMER), May 21, 2015.
3. Goldberg, Joseph, MD. "Somatic Symptom Disorder," WebMD, February 9, 2017.

Chapter 35 | Substance-Use Disorder

IS DRUG ADDICTION A MENTAL ILLNESS?

Yes, because addiction changes the brain in fundamental ways, disturbing a person's normal hierarchy of needs and desires and substituting new priorities connected with procuring and using the drug. The resulting compulsive behaviors that override the ability to control impulses despite the consequences are similar to hallmarks of other mental illnesses. In fact, the *Diagnostic and Statistical Manual of Mental Disorders* (DSM), which is the definitive resource of diagnostic criteria for all mental disorders, includes criteria for drug-use disorder(s), distinguishing between two types: drug abuse and drug dependence. By comparison, the criteria for drug abuse hinge on the harmful consequences of repeated use but do not include the compulsive use, tolerance (i.e., needing higher doses to achieve the same effect), or withdrawal (i.e., symptoms that occur when use is stopped) that can be signs of addiction.

HOW COMMON ARE COMORBID DRUG USE AND OTHER MENTAL DISORDERS?

Many people who regularly abuse drugs are also diagnosed with mental disorders and vice versa. The high prevalence of this

This chapter contains text excerpted from the following sources: Text beginning with the heading "Is Drug Addiction a Mental Illness?" is excerpted from "Comorbidity: Addiction and Other Mental Illnesses," National Institute on Drug Abuse (NIDA), September 2010. Reviewed August 2020; Text under the heading "Common Mechanistic Links between AUDs and Mood and Anxiety Disorders" is excerpted from "Focus on: Comorbid Mental Health Disorders," National Institute on Alcohol Abuse and Alcoholism (NIAAA), 2010. Reviewed August 2020.

comorbidity has been documented in multiple national population surveys since the 1980s. Data show that persons diagnosed with mood or anxiety disorders are about twice as likely to suffer also from a drug-use disorder (abuse or dependence) compared with respondents in general. The same is true for those diagnosed with an antisocial syndrome, such as antisocial personality or conduct disorder. Similarly, persons diagnosed with drug disorders are roughly twice as likely to suffer also from mood and anxiety disorders.

Gender is also a factor in the specific patterns of observed comorbidities. For example, the overall rates of abuse and dependence for most drugs tend to be higher among males than females. Further, males are more likely to suffer from antisocial personality disorder, while women have higher rates of mood and anxiety disorders, all of which are risk factors for substance abuse.

COMMON MECHANISTIC LINKS BETWEEN ALCOHOL-USE DISORDER(S) AND MOOD AND ANXIETY DISORDERS

A common thread linking alcohol-use disorder(s) (AUDs) with other comorbid mental-health disorders such as depression and posttraumatic stress disorder (PTSD) is the role that stress plays in precipitating and maintaining these disorders. Below is a brief sketch of how a better understanding of the irregularities in the brain's stress-reward systems might help elucidate the interrelationships among AUDs and some stress-related psychiatric disorders.

Components of the Stress Response

When an organism perceives a threat or when there is a challenge to its normal state (i.e., homeostasis), outgoing signals from multiple parts of the brain funnel input to the hypothalamus. The paraventricular nucleus (PVN) within the hypothalamus contains nerve cells (i.e., neurons) responsible for secreting corticotropin releasing hormone (CRH) and the hormone arginine vasopressin (AVP). The stress induced release of CRH and AVP into the portal circulation triggers the release of adrenocorticotropic hormone (ACTH) from the anterior pituitary gland, which, in humans, ultimately stimulates the production of cortisol (i.e., the stress hormone) from the adrenal cortex. A regulatory system is in place to turn off the endocrine stress response. Thus, the hormonal response to stress is mediated through the limbic-hypothalamic-pituitary-adrenal (LHPA) axis.

In addition to this hypothalamic-pituitary-adrenal (HPA) neuroendocrine stress axis, a parallel extrahypothalamic CRH (eCRH) brain stress system exists. This circuitry has its roots in a portion of the brain called the "extended amygdalae." The amygdalae (singular amygdala) are almond-shaped groups of neurons located deep within the medial temporal lobes of the brain. They encompass several nuclei, or structures in the central nervous system (CNS), including the central, lateral, and basal nuclei. The extended amygdala is composed of a group of structures, including the central nucleus of the amygdala (CeA) and the bed nucleus of stria terminalis (BNST), a group of neurons in the forebrain. CRH is produced by neurons in the CeA, the BNST, and the brainstem. This eCRH system helps mediate behavioral responses to stress and controls the sympathetic nervous system response to stressors. It is important to note that although the HPA-CRH and extended amygdalar-eCRH stress circuits are interconnected, the latter system can act independent of the HPA axis. Several different chemicals that transmit impulses between neurons (i.e., neurotransmitters) regulate the CRH systems in the brain, but interactions between norepinephrine and CRH in the region of the locus coeruleus (a nucleus in the brainstem) are believed to be particularly relevant to alcoholism and certain stress-related psychiatric disorders, such as major depression and PTSD. Other key neurotransmitters regulating these stress-reward circuits—which are likely to play a role in comorbid alcoholism and stress-related disorders—are serotonin, endogenous opiates, γ-aminobutyric acid (GABA), and glutamate.

Chronic Alcohol Disrupts the Hypothalamic-Pituitary-Adrenal Stress Response

It has been hypothesized that a key interface between the brain's stress systems and reward circuits lies in the region of the extended amygdala. It is here that the positive reinforcing effects of drugs, including alcohol, and the negative reinforcing effects of these agents are believed to intersect, with the CRH systems playing a critical modulatory role in this interaction.

In both experimental animals and humans, alcohol intoxication results in the release of CRH and activation of the HPA axis. Based on evidence from studies with rodents, it appears that these stress-activating effects may be greater in women than men. Although it might seem counterintuitive to consider that consumption of alcohol increases the brain's and body's stress hormone levels, it is likely that the brain adapts to repeated bouts of heavy drinking by downregulating responsive elements in the stress circuitry, and it is this process (i.e., neuroadaptation) that characterizes aspects of the addiction process.

Effects of Alcohol Withdrawal on the Stress Response

Alcohol's activation of the stress systems is even more profound during acute withdrawal. Studies in experimental animals and humans show marked increases in brain CRH levels and plasma ACTH and cortisol concentrations, respectively, in the hours and days following the last exposure to alcohol. This hyperactivation of the brain's stress system is accompanied by anxiety-like behaviors in experimental animals and depressed mood in humans. Furthermore, studies in rodents demonstrate that administering drugs that block CRH activity in the CeA (i.e., CRH antagonists) can block these aversive withdrawal effects.

According to Koob and LeMoal's theory, the compulsive stage of alcohol dependence is produced, in part, by alcohol-seeking behaviors to relieve a "negative affect state," which, according to these authors, may be a hallmark of the protracted abstinence syndrome. Furthermore, the neurobiological underpinnings of this negative emotional state originate in the extended amygdala and are mediated through interactions among the CRH, GABAergic, and norepinephrine systems. A final piece of the theory postulates that alcohol and other drug addiction is marked by an ongoing adaptation (or allostatic change) in these stress-reward systems, meaning that alcohol dependent individuals have adjusted their biological set points and have become more sensitive to stressors and more prone to stress-induced relapse to alcohol. Indeed, in the days and weeks following the acute withdrawal period, the HPA axis remains dysregulated in alcoholics. However, during this subacute or protracted withdrawal phase, the system is typically blunted. That is, when challenged by a variety of stressors, the endocrine response typically is lower than normal. A few studies have linked these abnormal stress responses with the individual's risk of relapse to drinking. With lengthier abstinence, however, the HPA axis response to stress appears to normalize.

Overlapping Mechanisms with Other Stress-Related Disorders

Stress is known to contribute to the development of alcoholism in at-risk individuals and to the maintenance of the disease through stress-induced relapse. It also is a well-known precipitant of stress-related psychiatric disorders such as major depressive disorder (MDD) and PTSD. In fact, the principle of allostasis, which plays a central role in Koob and LeMoal's theories on addiction also plays an integral role in McEwen and Wingfield's and other scientists' perspectives on the development of stress-related mood and anxiety disorders. In those hypotheses, chronic stress produces an "allostatic state" (e.g., chronic elevations in steroid hormones [i.e., glucocorticoids]) that can damage brain structures (e.g., the hippocampus, which inhibits the HPA) and cause other compensatory neuroadaptive changes, such as changes to the neurotransmitter binding molecules (i.e., receptors) that lead to desensitization. Cumulatively, the dysregulated stress responses produce an "allostatic load" on the organism that contributes to tissue damage, cognitive deficits, and chronic illnesses such as cardiovascular disease (CVD).

Just as alcoholics display changes in HPA axis function that vary as a function of disease state, people with stress-related psychiatric disorders such as MDD and PTSD manifest dysregulated HPA axis responsivity.

Given that MDD, PTSD, and AUDs so frequently overlap, the challenge confronting researchers in the next decade and beyond is to tease out whether the pattern of altered stress responses seen in comorbid patients shows evidence of greater or lesser dysregulation compared with patients with only one disorder. It is possible that alcohol may exacerbate or counterbalance stress system abnormalities associated with these disorders in the absence of alcoholism.

Chapter 36 | Suicidal Ideation

The combinations of various factors, such as sociological, psychological, cultural, and economic effects, are the major reasons for suicide. The widely established suicide-related nomenclature includes suicide attempts, nonfatal suicide attempts, and suicidal ideation. The intention and expression of killing oneself is known as "suicidal ideation." Every year 10–20 million people attempt suicide, and nearly a million die. Mood disorders and personality disorders (in particular borderline personality disorder) are the most commonly associated medical conditions with suicide, along with the rising impact of anxiety disorders on suicide.

Psychiatric conditions are one of the key risk factors for suicidality, with up to 95 percent of people suffering from one or more conditions. The known risk factors for suicidal attempts include affective disorders, drug abuse, depressive disorders, other behavioral conditions, and psychiatric disorders. Notably, the probability of attempted suicide is 20 and 10 times higher for bipolar affective disorder and schizophrenia, respectively. A corresponding decline in the suicide rate is identified where a successful diagnosis of mental conditions are completed, indicating that unresolved psychological morbidity is an factor of elevated suicidal risk in itself.

While anxiety and depression are two separate conditions with different symptoms and treatments, it is not uncommon for someone to experience both disorders simultaneously. Suicidal ideation is one of the most concerning symptoms a person dealing with anxiety and depression can exhibit. Anxiety and depression are highly treatable disorders with outstandingly high efficacy rates for therapies. Patients of anxiety disorders are at high risk of suicidal ideation, regardless of whether the suicidal ideation is related to anxiety symptoms or co-occurring illnesses themselves.

CAUSES OF SUICIDAL IDEATION

Suicidal ideation can occur when a person thinks they cannot deal with a stressful situation any longer. It may be due to:
- Financial issues
- Sexual harassment
- Toxic relationships
- Severe illness
- Loss of a loved one
- Unemployment
- History of mental-health problems
- Family history of violence
- Sexuality not being accepted such as being lesbian, gay, bisexual, or transgender (LGBT)
- Being addicted to drugs or alcohol

Apart from the causes, certain mental-health disorders can also be a triggering factor for committing suicide or having suicidal thoughts, such as:
- Schizophrenia
- Bipolar disorder
- Posttraumatic stress disorder (PTSD)
- Anorexia nervosa
- Generalized anxiety disorder (GAD)
- Gender identity disorder
- Depression
- Genetic factors

SYMPTOMS OF SUICIDAL IDEATION

A majority of people with suicidal ideation keep their emotions and intentions a secret and show no signs. The common signs and symptoms that are exhibited by people having suicidal thoughts are:

- Talking about death and dying
- Constantly criticizing life
- Feeling extreme emotional pain
- Exhibiting violent behavior
- Feeling hopeless, guilty, or ashamed
- Being agitated
- Change in routine and personality
- Started consuming drugs or alcohol
- Talking about being a burden to people
- Possessing ammunition or drugs that could be lethal
- Engaging in risky behavior (reckless driving)
- Lack of concentration in daily tasks
- Pacing around a room, constant murmuring, or shaking of hands
- Saying goodbye as if it were the last time

REDUCING THE RISKS OF SUICIDAL IDEATION

Suicidal thoughts can be easily reduced or prevented by attempting the following:

- Avoiding illegal drugs and alcohol
- Doing exercise and other physical activities
- Eating a healthy, well-balanced diet
- Staying connected socially
- Getting proper and sufficient sleep
- Removing dangerous items such as guns, knives, drugs, chemicals, and other lethal items from home
- Talking to family members about how you feel

Helping a Friend or Loved One from Suicidal Tendencies

- Talking or asking close ones on how they feel, whether they have any negative thoughts or so
- Encouraging and talking to them to do something new in life
- Being there for them and listening to what they have to say
- Indulging them in activities and programs

- Staying in touch with them after they have been in a crisis, discharged from care facilities or been in a major problem
- Connecting them with a trustable person or new friends
- The National Suicide Prevention Lifeline's number—800-273-TALK (800-273-8255)—can be saved in case of any emergency. The Crisis Text Line is 741741.

References

1. Hocauglu, Cicek. "Anxiety Disorder and Suicide: Psychiatric Interventions," Intechopen, September 9, 2015.
2. "Suicide and Prevention," Anxiety and Depression Association of America (ADAA), September 6, 2016.
3. Brazier, Yvette. "What Are Suicidal Thoughts," Medical News Today, February 13, 2018.
4. Nepon, Josh; Bolton, James. "The Relationship Between Anxiety Disorders and Suicide Attempts," National Center for Biotechnology Information (NCBI), March 16, 2010.

Part 5 | Lifestyle Modifications for Mental Health and Well-Being

Chapter 37 | **Emotional Wellness Toolkit**

How you feel can affect your ability to carry out everyday activities, your relationships, and your overall mental health. How you react to your experiences and feelings can change over time. Emotional wellness is the ability to successfully handle life's stresses and adapt to change and difficult times. Here are six strategies for improving your emotional health.

BRIGHTEN YOUR OUTLOOK

People who are emotionally well, experts say, have fewer negative emotions and are able to bounce back from difficulties faster. This quality is called "resilience." Another sign of emotional wellness is being able to hold onto positive emotions longer and appreciate the good times.

To develop a more positive mindset:

- **Remember your good deeds.** Give yourself credit for the good things you do for others each day.
- **Forgive yourself.** Everyone makes mistakes. Learn from what went wrong, but do not dwell on it.
- **Spend more time with your friends.** Surround yourself with positive, healthy people.
- **Explore your beliefs about the meaning and purpose of life.** Think about how to guide your life by the principles that are important to you.

This chapter includes text excerpted from "Emotional Wellness Toolkit," National Institutes of Health (NIH), December 10, 2018.

- **Develop healthy physical habits.** Healthy eating, physical activity, and regular sleep can improve your physical and mental health.

REDUCE STRESS

Everyone feels stressed from time to time. Stress can give you a rush of energy when it is needed most. But, if the stress lasts a long time—a condition known as "chronic stress"—those "high-alert" changes become harmful rather than helpful. Learning healthy ways to cope with stress can also boost your resilience.

To help manage stress:
- **Get enough sleep.**
- **Exercise regularly.** Just 30 minutes a day of walking can boost mood and reduce stress.
- **Build a social support network.**
- **Set priorities.** Decide what must get done and what can wait. Say no to new tasks if they are putting you into overload.
- **Think positive.** Note what you have accomplished at the end of the day, not what you have failed to do.
- **Try relaxation methods.** Mindfulness, meditation, yoga, or tai chi may help.
- **Seek help.** Talk to a mental-health professional if you feel unable to cope, have suicidal thoughts, or use drugs or alcohol to cope.

GET QUALITY SLEEP

To fit in everything we want to do in our day, we often sacrifice sleep. But, sleep affects both mental and physical health. It is vital to your well-being. When you are tired, you cannot function at your best. Sleep helps you think more clearly, have quicker reflexes, and focus better. Take steps to make sure you regularly get a good night's sleep.

To get better quality sleep:
- Go to bed at the same time each night and get up the same time each morning.

- Sleep in a dark, quiet, comfortable environment.
- Exercise daily (but not right before bedtime).
- Limit the use of electronics before bed.
- Relax before bedtime. A warm bath or reading might help.
- Avoid alcohol and stimulants such as caffeine late in the day.
- Avoid nicotine.
- Consult a healthcare professional if you have ongoing sleep problems.

COPE WITH LOSS

When someone you love dies, your world changes. There is no right or wrong way to mourn. Although the death of a loved one can feel overwhelming, most people can make it through the grieving process with the support of family and friends. Learn healthy ways to help you through difficult times.

To help cope with loss:

- **Take care of yourself.** Try to eat right, exercise, and get enough sleep. Avoid bad habits—like smoking or drinking alcohol—that can put your health at risk.
- **Talk to caring friends.** Let others know when you want to talk.
- **Find a grief support group**. It might help to talk with others who are also grieving.
- **Do not make major changes right away**. Wait a while before making big decisions like moving or changing jobs.
- **Talk to your doctor** if you are having trouble with everyday activities.
- **Consider additional support.** Sometimes short-term talk therapy can help.
- **Be patient.** Mourning takes time. It is common to have roller-coaster emotions for a while.

STRENGTHEN SOCIAL CONNECTIONS

Social connections might help protect health and lengthen life. Scientists are finding that our links to others can have powerful effects on our health—both emotionally and physically. Whether with romantic partners, family, friends, neighbors, or others, social connections can influence our biology and well-being.

To build healthy support systems:

- Build strong relationships with your kids.
- Get active and share good habits with family and friends.
- If you are a family caregiver, ask for help from others.
- Join a group focused on a favorite hobby such as reading, hiking, or painting.
- Take a class to learn something new.
- Volunteer for things you care about in your community, such as a community garden, school, library, or place of worship.
- Travel to different places and meet new people.

BE MINDFUL

The concept of mindfulness is simple. This ancient practice is about being completely aware of what is happening in the present—of all, that is going on inside and all that is happening around you. It means not living your life on "autopilot." Becoming a more mindful person requires commitment and practice. Here are some tips to help you get started.

To be more mindful:

- **Take some deep breaths.** Breathe in through your nose to a count of 4, hold for 1 second, and then exhale through the mouth to a count of 5. Repeat often.
- **Enjoy a stroll.** As you walk, notice your breath and the sights and sounds around you. As thoughts and worries enter your mind, note them but then return to the present.
- **Practice mindful eating**. Be aware of taste, textures, and flavors in each bite, and listen to your body when you are hungry and full.
- **Find mindfulness resources in your local community**, including yoga and meditation classes, mindfulness-based stress reduction programs, and books.

Chapter 38 | Diet and Physical Activity

Chapter Contents

Section 38.1 | Healthy Eating and Physical Activity for Mental-Health Benefits

This section includes text excerpted from "Supporting Clients to Make Healthy Food Choices and Increase Physical Activity," Substance Abuse and Mental Health Services Administration (SAMHSA), September 2014. Reviewed August 2020.

More than one-third of adults in the United States are obese (34.9%). Obesity, often due to preventable behaviors, is a contributing factor of many leading causes of death, including heart disease, diabetes, stroke, and some types of cancer. Rates of obesity are increasing across all socioeconomic and education levels, with the average American gaining 1 to 2 pounds per year, every year.

Individuals with behavioral health and other chronic health conditions are even more at risk for weight-related death and disability. Prevalence studies find that individuals with behavioral health conditions are overweight or obese at double the rate found in the general population. For this reason, excess weight among persons with behavioral health conditions has been deemed an epidemic within an epidemic.

Specific psychiatric disorders and the use of many psychiatric medications are directly tied to weight issues. For example, depression is more common among people who are obese than those who have a healthy weight. Research indicates that obesity may increase risk of depression by as much as 55 percent, but that depression also increases risk of obesity by 58 percent. Also, some individuals diagnosed with schizophrenia are sedentary over three-quarters of their waking day (81%), contributing greatly to excess weight.

Weight management can be difficult for anyone, but persons with behavioral health conditions face additional barriers to sustained weight loss. Weight gain is a common side effect of many psychiatric medications and associated metabolic syndrome. Individuals who begin psychiatric medications at an earlier age (less than 24 years of age), and who remain on the medication for at least five years, are more likely to be obese. Moreover, studies indicate that individuals with diagnoses such as schizophrenia engage in low levels of physical exercise and are more likely to consume high-calorie foods that have insufficient nutrient value.

In addition to increased risk of death and disability associated with being overweight, individuals who are obese also face increased stigma and discrimination from the general public, employers, and healthcare providers: "Weight bias translates into inequalities in employment settings, healthcare facilities, and educational institutions, often due to widespread negative stereotypes that persons who are overweight and obese are lazy, unmotivated, lacking in self-discipline, less competent, noncompliant, and sloppy.

MAKING HEALTHY FOOD CHOICES

As defined by the U.S. Department of Agriculture (USDA), patients often experience:

- Food deserts, which are low-income communities with limited access to healthy foods like fresh fruits and vegetables
- Food insecurity, the limited or uncertain availability of nutritionally adequate and safe foods, or the ability to acquire acceptable foods in socially acceptable ways

A common barrier to making healthy food choices include some patients' limited financial resources. Healthy food is often more expensive than processed food. While convenient, processed foods are often high in salt, fat, and carbohydrates. Individuals in psychiatric hospitals or congregate living settings may have limited access to a kitchen or may only be provided with high-calorie foods that are low in nutrients. Also, when patients do have access to kitchens for personal cooking, many have never learned how to prepare healthy meals. For many, eating is a way to cope with stress, boredom, or other negative mood states and patients may need to develop new constructive coping strategies. Moreover, patients may live in areas that may be unsafe for physical activity, or other community resources are scarce.

Weight gain is due to a combination of biological and psychosocial factors, however, eating a healthy, balanced diet and being physically active is essential for achieving a healthy weight and feeling well. Popular exercise programs often over-promise quick-fix "miracle workouts" or are not intuitively modifiable to meet all fitness levels. And it is also easy to become sidetracked by the latest weight loss and exercise fads, diets, and procedures.

Providers can communicate a number of other measurable benefits to regular physical activity. Moderate physical activity decreases risk of cardiovascular disease (CVD), improves mood in people living with depression, increases emotional health for people diagnosed with schizophrenia, improves cognitive functions in those living with dementia, and improves self-esteem in children and adolescents.

Many providers may feel uncomfortable discussing a patient's weight or are less willing to engage patients on a topic they feel may be too challenging. As healthcare providers, it is important to have empathy for people who are overweight or obese and constructively support their efforts to lose weight. Changing nutritional and exercise habits is difficult and, without support, failure is common.

Making lifestyle changes takes motivation and new skills which providers can effectively promote. It is critical that providers support patients to create achievable, person-centered goals, and expectations for sustained lifestyle changes. For instance, while weight loss bolsters motivation to persist in health behavior change strategies, failure to lose weight is associated with reverting back to unhealthy habits. Providers can be of best help to patients by supporting them to avoid time-limited strategies (such as diets) and instead supporting them to create person-centered wellness goals that they might permanently integrate into their lives. These are "small wins," such as progressively drinking less soda or a daily practice of attending to emotional well-being through journaling.

While physical activity and dietary needs must be tailored to patients health status and physical ability, increased physical activity in combination with a balanced diet carries few risks and is nearly always advisable. For some patients, aerobic activities might be incrementally increased walking or chair-based activities. Whether healthy eating and/or increased physical activity is the patient's primary goal, providers can actively engage patients in discussions of personal wellness, assist them to set achievable goals, and then monitor progress over time.

KEEP IT SIMPLE AND EFFECTIVE

The most powerful tool a provider has is their relationship with their patients and the most effective healthy living strategies focus on increasing motivation to change; achievable, person-centered goal setting; and referral to evidence-based services. It is important that providers adopt a patient's-led approach, which focuses on individual concerns and specific reasons or benefits of current behaviors.

Patients may not want to initially discuss weight and physical activity. Meet the patient where they are and focus on their strengths. Allow patients to express what they feel are their primary physical and emotional health issues first and then, if appropriate, identify ways to individually introduce healthy eating and increased physical activity based on their strengths and supports into the treatment dialogue. An important strategy for meeting patients where they are is to invite open discussion of how their community and family influences their eating and physical activity habits.

The 5 A's model of intervention (Ask, Advise, Assess, Assist, and Arrange) is a practical structure for addressing many wellness issues, including healthy eating and physical activity, follow-up, and community referrals.

Section 38.2 | The Emotional Benefits of Physical Activity and Exercise

This section includes text excerpted from "Managing Stress with Exercise," Federal Occupational Health (FOH), U.S. Department of Health and Human Services (HHS), 2004. Reviewed August 2020.

Stress can make you feel drained, anxious, even depressed. And while there are several ways to manage runaway stress, none is as enjoyable and effective as a regular exercise routine. "Numerous studies have shown exercise provides excellent stress-relieving benefits," says Cedric Bryant, chief exercise physiologist for the American Council on exercise in San Diego.

HOW IT WORKS

Exercise causes the brain to release endorphins, opium-like substances that ease pain, and produce a sense of comfort and euphoria. It also encourages the nerve cells in the brain to secrete other neurotransmitters that improve mood.

Deficiencies of these substances have been linked to symptoms of depression, anxiety, impulsiveness, aggression, and increased appetite. According to a study published in the *Archives of Internal Medicine*, exercise increases the levels of these natural antidepressants.

According to the National Institutes of Health (NIH), exercise also improves people's ability to relax and sleep, promotes self-esteem, and enhances energy, concentration, and memory.

STRESS-REDUCTION MOVES

The following guidelines can help you find activities likely to be effective for you:

- **Choose an exercise you enjoy.** "It is important to choose activities that are accessible and feasible for you to do regularly," says Bryant. "You also need to determine if you want to play competitive sports, such as basketball or tennis, or if you would rather do non competitive activities such as walking, bicycling, or taking an aerobics class."
- **Exercise every day if you can.** The U.S. Surgeon General's Report on Physical Activity and Health recommends 30 minutes of activity on most, if not all, days of the week.
- **Consider mind–body activities.** In yoga and tai chi, your mind relaxes progressively as your body increases its amount of muscular work. "These forms of exercise are effective for honing stress management and relaxation skills," says Bryant.

Controlling stress ultimately comes down to making time to exercise. Physical activity provides an enjoyable and effective way to cope with life's troubles as it promotes lasting strength and empowerment.

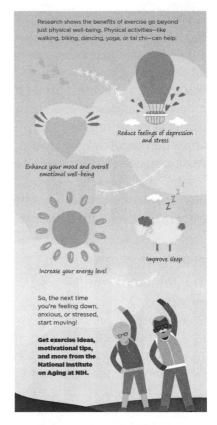

Figure 38.1. Emotional Benefits of Exercise
(Source: National Institute on Aging (NIA),
National Institutes of Health (NIH))

Section 38.3 | **Walking to Wellness**

This section includes text excerpted from "Walking to Wellness," Mental Illness Research, Education and Clinical Centers (MIRECC), U.S. Department of Veterans Affairs (VA), December 2015. Reviewed August 2020.

HOW CAN WALKING TO WELLNESS HELP YOU?

A brisk walk or other physical activity can improve your mood quickly and help you feel better for up to several hours. Regular walking can also help reduce anxiety and depression symptoms over long periods of time.

If you are already active, the suggestions here may help you enjoy exercise more and get more emotional benefit. If you have not been doing any regular physical activity, the activities are designed to help you start regular walking during the next four weeks. You may choose a different kind of exercise or progress at a different pace that is better for you. The Mental Illness Research, Education and Clinical Centers (MIRECC) especially recommends walking because it is easy and safe for most people and there is substantial scientific evidence that walking is good for physical and mental health.

SOME BASIC FACTS: HOW DOES PHYSICAL ACTIVITY AFFECT HEALTH?

Let us begin with a look at why "exercise is medicine." Some of these benefits can be felt almost immediately, but others build gradually after several weeks of regular activity. Making time to be active almost every day will bring you slowly and surely to the most benefit from your efforts.

WHAT KIND OF EXERCISE AND HOW MUCH IS NECESSARY?

Many people want to know "What do I have to do?" and "How much exercise is necessary?" The MIRECC now has a lot of information from scientific research to answer those questions and help you plan your exercise time in the best way for emotional, as well as physical health.

Health experts say the amount of exercise that most adults need is a total of about 30 minutes of moderate endurance exercise most days. Endurance exercise includes walking, jogging, swimming, cycling, and other activities with repeated muscle movement that you can do for extended periods of time.

How Hard Do You Have to Work Out?

Moderate exercise is hard enough so you feel your breathing increase and start to sweat. You can still carry on a conversation, but you do not have enough breath to sing out loud. As you gain experience, activity will get easier to do and you can do more at the same level of effort. Exercise is hard or vigorous if you are breathing hard enough so that you cannot talk or sing.

A total of about 30 minutes per day of moderate endurance activity seems to be enough to improve or maintain emotional and mental health as well as physical health for most adults. This may not be the right goal for you.

HOW MUCH EXERCISE IS BEST FOR YOU?

Spending a total of 30 minutes a day on most days walking or doing other moderate exercise may seem impossible. You may feel that you are too busy, or that you could never make yourself do it because you do not like exercise or getting sweaty. Perhaps you have a health condition such as pain that limits your activity. In these situations, it is helpful to remember that you can exercise for shorter periods of time several times during the day. At least 10 minutes at a time seems best for experiencing immediate emotional benefits from exercise, but every minute counts for overall health.

Another way to think about it is that every step that you take will move you toward greater wellness. The scientific evidence shows that any activity is better than none. You can choose a plan that works for you.

If you have not been exercising regularly, be smart and safe—give yourself time to ease gradually into more activity. It may take several weeks of regular activity to feel comfortable with a moderate walking speed and effort.

HOW DO YOU SET EXERCISE GOALS?

It can be hard to follow through and actually accomplish a wellness goal. If you ever made a New Year's resolution and then did not keep it, you know that wanting to do something is not always enough to build and sustain the motivation needed to accomplish the goal.

There are some strategies that people can use to be successful in achieving a goal they feel is important to them.

First, it helps to be very specific about what it is that you want to do. Can you imagine yourself going for a 10 minute walk with the purpose of taking care of yourself? Where would you like to walk? What time of the day? What will you wear? Will someone be walking with you?

Planning the details of what you want to do will help you understand whether your plan is workable. This can also help you identify problems that could get in the way. For example, if you want to walk outdoors, what will you do if it is raining? Or if you plan to walk with someone, what will be your new plan if that person is not able to go with you?

The MIRECC recommends that you write down your plans and include those details. You will notice that the last entry on that page is a confidence rating. Be honest with yourself when you rate your confidence in achieving your goal.

Chapter 39 | Avoiding Caffeine, Nicotine, and Alcohol

Chapter Contents

Section 39.1 | Cutting Back on Caffeine

This section contains text excerpted from the following sources: Text beginning with the heading "What Is Caffeine?" is excerpted from "Caffeine," MedlinePlus, National Institutes of Health (NIH), April 14, 2020; Text under the heading "Tips to Avoid Caffeine" is excerpted from "The Buzz on Caffeine," National Institute on Drug Abuse (NIDA) for Teens, June 25, 2014. Reviewed August 2020.

WHAT IS CAFFEINE?

Caffeine is a bitter substance that occurs naturally in more than 60 plants including:

- Coffee beans
- Tea leaves
- Kola nuts, which are used to flavor soft drink colas
- Cacao pods, which are used to make chocolate products

There is also synthetic (human-made) caffeine, which is added to some medicines, foods, and drinks. For example, some pain relievers, cold medicines, and over-the-counter (OTC) medicines for alertness contain synthetic caffeine. So do energy drinks and "energy-boosting" gums and snacks.

Most people consume caffeine from drinks. The amounts of caffeine in different drinks can vary a lot, but it is generally:

- An 8-ounce cup of coffee: 95–200 mg
- A 12-ounce can of cola: 35–45 mg
- An 8-ounce energy drink: 70–100 mg
- An 8-ounce cup of tea: 14–60 mg

WHAT ARE CAFFEINE'S EFFECTS ON THE BODY?

Caffeine has many effects on your body's metabolism. It:

- Stimulates your central nervous system, which can make you feel more awake and give you a boost of energy
- Is a diuretic, meaning that it helps your body get rid of extra salt and water by urinating more
- Increases the release of acid in your stomach, sometimes leading to an upset stomach or heartburn

- May interfere with the absorption of calcium in the body
- Increases your blood pressure

Within one hour of eating or drinking caffeine, it reaches its peak level in your blood. You may continue to feel the effects of caffeine for four to six hours.

WHAT ARE THE SIDE EFFECTS FROM TOO MUCH CAFFEINE?

For most people, it is not harmful to consume up to 400mg of caffeine a day. If you do eat or drink too much caffeine, it can cause health problems, such as:

- Restlessness and shakiness
- Insomnia
- Headaches
- Dizziness
- Rapid or abnormal heart rhythm
- Dehydration
- Anxiety
- Dependency, so you need to take more of it to get the same results

Some people are more sensitive to the effects of caffeine than others.

WHO SHOULD AVOID OR LIMIT CAFFEINE?

You should check with your healthcare provider about whether you should limit or avoid caffeine if you:

- Are pregnant, since caffeine passes through the placenta to your baby
- Are breastfeeding, since a small amount of caffeine that you consume is passed along to your baby
- Have sleep disorders, including insomnia
- Have migraines or other chronic headaches
- Have anxiety
- Have gastroesophageal reflux disease (GERD) or ulcers

- Have fast or irregular heart rhythms
- Have high blood pressure
- Take certain medicines or supplements, including stimulants, certain antibiotics, asthma medicines, and heart medicines. Check with your healthcare provider about whether there might be interactions between caffeine and any medicines and supplements that you take.
- Are a child or teen. Neither should have as much caffeine as adults. Children can be especially sensitive to the effects of caffeine.

WHAT IS CAFFEINE WITHDRAWAL?

If you have been consuming caffeine on a regular basis and then suddenly stop, you may have caffeine withdrawal. Symptoms can include:
- Headaches
- Drowsiness
- Irritability
- Nausea
- Difficulty concentrating

These symptoms usually go away after a couple of days.

TIPS TO AVOID CAFFEINE

Drinking a cup of coffee, or eating a bar of chocolate, is usually not a big deal. But, there are alternatives to caffeine if you are looking for an energy burst but do not want to get that jittery feeling caffeine sometimes causes. Here are a few alternatives you can try to feel energized without overdoing the caffeine:
- **Sleep.** This may sound obvious, but getting enough sleep is important.
- **Eat regularly.** When you do not eat, your glucose (sugar) levels drop, making you feel drained. Some people find it helpful to eat four or five smaller meals throughout the day instead of fewer big meals.

- **Drink enough water.** Since our bodies are more than two-thirds H_2O, we need at least 64 ounces of water a day.
- **Take a walk.** If you are feeling drained in the middle of the day, it helps to move around. Do sit-ups or jumping jacks. Go outside for a brisk walk or ride your bike.

Section 39.2 | Smoking Cessation and Mental-Health Benefits

This section includes text excerpted from "How to Handle Withdrawal Symptoms and Triggers when You Decide to Quit Smoking," National Cancer Institute (NCI), October 29, 2010. Reviewed August 2020.

Quitting smoking may cause short-term problems, especially for those who have smoked heavily for many years. These temporary changes can result in withdrawal symptoms.

Common withdrawal symptoms associated with quitting include the following:

- Nicotine cravings
- Anger, frustration, and irritability
- Anxiety
- Depression
- Weight gain

Studies have shown that about half of smokers report experiencing at least four withdrawal symptoms (such as anger, anxiety, or depression) when they quit. People have reported other symptoms, including dizziness, increased dreaming, and headaches.

The good news is that there is much you can do to reduce cravings and manage common withdrawal symptoms. Even without medication, withdrawal symptoms, and other problems subside over time. It may also help to know that withdrawal symptom are usually worst during the first week after quitting. From that point on, the intensity usually drops over the first month. However, everyone is different, and some people have withdrawal symptoms for several months after quitting.

AVOIDING SMOKING TRIGGERS

In addition to nicotine cravings, reminders in your daily life of times when you used to smoke may trigger you to smoke. Triggers are the moods, feelings, places, or things you do in your daily life that turn on your desire to smoke.

Triggers may include any of the following:

- Being around smokers
- Starting the day
- Feeling stressed
- Being in a car
- Drinking coffee or tea
- Enjoying a meal
- Drinking an alcoholic beverage
- Feeling bored

Knowing your triggers helps you stay in control because you can choose to avoid them or keep your mind distracted and busy when you cannot avoid them.

NICOTINE CRAVINGS

As a smoker, you get used to having a certain level of nicotine in your body. You control that level by how much you smoke, how deeply you inhale the smoke, and the kind of tobacco you use. When you quit, cravings develop when your body wants nicotine. It takes time to break free from nicotine addiction. Also, when you see people smoking or are around other triggers, you may get nicotine cravings. Cravings are real. They are not just in your imagination. At the same time, your mood may change, and your heart rate and blood pressure may go up.

The urge to smoke will come and go. Cravings usually last only a very brief period of time. Cravings usually begin within an hour or two after you have your last cigarette, peak for several days, and may last several weeks. As the days pass, the cravings will get farther apart. Occasional mild cravings may last for six months.

Here are some tips for managing cravings:

- Remind yourself that they will pass.

- Avoid situations and activities that you used to associate with smoking.
- As a substitute for smoking, try chewing on carrots, pickles, apples, celery, sugarless gum, or hard candy. Keeping your mouth busy may stop the psychological need to smoke.
- Try this exercise: Take a deep breath through your nose and blow out slowly through your mouth. Repeat ten times.
- Ask your doctor about nicotine replacement products or other medications.

DEALING WITH ANGER, FRUSTRATION, AND IRRITABILITY

After you quit smoking, you may feel edgy and short-tempered, and you may want to give up on tasks more quickly than usual. You may be less tolerant of others and get into more arguments.

Studies have found that the most common negative feelings associated with quitting are feelings of anger, frustration, and irritability. These negative feelings peak within one week of quitting and may last 2 to 4 weeks.

QUITTING AND ANXIETY

Within 24 hours of quitting smoking, you may feel tense and agitated. You may feel a tightness in your muscles—especially around the neck and shoulders. Studies have found that anxiety is one of the most common negative feelings associated with quitting. If anxiety occurs, it builds over the first 3 days after quitting and may last two weeks.

Here are some tips for managing anxiety:
- Remind yourself that anxiety will pass with time.
- Set aside some quiet time every morning and evening—a time when you can be alone in a quiet environment.
- Engage in physical activity, such as taking a walk.
- Reduce caffeine by limiting or avoiding coffee, soda, and tea.

- Try meditation or other relaxation techniques such as getting a massage, soaking in a hot bath, or breathing deeply through your nose and out through your mouth for ten breaths.
- Ask your doctor about nicotine replacement products or other medications.

DEPRESSION AFTER QUITTING

It is normal to feel sad for a period of time after you first quit smoking. If mild depression occurs, it will usually begin within the first day, continue for the first couple of weeks, and go away within a month.

Having a history of depression is associated with more severe withdrawal symptoms—including more severe depression. Some studies have found that many people with a history of major depression will have a new major depressive episode after quitting. However, in those with no history of depression, major depression after quitting is rare.

Many people have a strong urge to smoke when they feel depressed.

Here are some tips for managing depression:

- Call a friend and plan to have lunch or go to a movie, concert, or other pleasurable event.
- Identify your specific feelings at the time that you seem depressed. Are you actually feeling tired, lonely, bored, or hungry? Focus on and address these specific needs.
- Increase physical activity. This will help to improve your mood and lift your depression.
- Breathe deeply.
- Make a list of things that are upsetting to you and write down solutions for them.
- If depression continues for more than one month, see your doctor. Ask your doctor about prescription medications that may help you with depression.

Section 39.3 | **Benefits of Quitting Alcohol**

This section contains text excerpted from the following sources: Text in this section begins with excerpts from "Building Your Drink Refusal Skills," National Institute on Alcohol Abuse and Alcoholism (NIAAA), March 10, 2009. Reviewed August 2020; Text beginning with the heading "Plan Ahead to Stay in Control" is excerpted from "Handling Urges to Drink," National Institute on Alcohol Abuse and Alcoholism (NIAAA), March 10, 2009. Reviewed August 2020.

Even if you are committed to changing your drinking, "social pressure" to drink from friends or others can make it hard to cut back or quit. This section offers a recognize-avoid-cope approach commonly used in cognitive-behavioral therapy (CBT), which helps people to change unhelpful thinking patterns and reactions.

RECOGNIZE TWO TYPES OF PRESSURE

The first step is to become aware of the two different types of social pressure to drink alcohol—direct and indirect.

- **Direct social pressure** is when someone offers you a drink or an opportunity to drink.
- **Indirect social pressure** is when you feel tempted to drink just by being around others who are drinking—even if no one offers you a drink.

Take a moment to think about situations where you feel direct or indirect pressure to drink or to drink too much. Then, for each situation, choose some resistance strategies from below, or come up with your own.

AVOID PRESSURE WHEN POSSIBLE

For some situations, your best strategy may be avoiding them altogether. If you feel guilty about avoiding an event or turning down an invitation, remind yourself that you are not necessarily talking about "forever." When you have confidence in your resistance skills, you may decide to ease gradually into situations you now choose to avoid. In the meantime, you can stay connected with friends by suggesting alternate activities that do not involve drinking.

COPE WITH SITUATIONS YOU CANNOT AVOID
Know Your "No"

When you know alcohol will be served, it is important to have some resistance strategies lined up in advance. If you expect to be offered a drink, you will need to be ready to deliver a convincing "no thanks." Your goal is to be clear and firm, yet friendly and respectful. Avoid long explanations and vague excuses, as they tend to prolong the discussion and provide more of an opportunity to give in. Here are some other points to keep in mind:

- Do not hesitate, as that will give you the chance to think of reasons to go along.
- Look directly at the person and make eye contact.
- Keep your response short, clear, and simple.

The person offering you a drink may not know you are trying to cut down or stop, and her or his level of insistence may vary. It is a good idea to plan a series of responses in case the person persists, from a simple refusal to a more assertive reply. Consider a sequence such as this:

- No, thank you.
- No, thanks, I do not want to.
- You know, I am (cutting back/not drinking) now (to get healthier/to take care of myself/because my doctor said to). I would really appreciate it if you could help me out.

You can also try the "broken record" strategy. Each time the person makes a statement, you can simply repeat the same short, clear response. You might want to acknowledge some part of the person's points ("I hear you...") and then go back to your broken-record reply ("...but no thanks"). And if words fail, you can walk away.

Script and Practice Your "No"

Many people are surprised at how hard it can be to say no the first few times. You can build confidence by scripting and practicing your lines. First imagine the situation and the person who is offering the drink. Then write both what the person will say and

289

how you will respond, whether it is a broken record strategy (mentioned above) or your own unique approach. Rehearse it aloud to get comfortable with your phrasing and delivery. Also, consider asking a supportive person to role-play with you, someone who would offer realistic pressure to drink and honest feedback about your responses. Whether you practice through made-up or real-world experiences, you will learn as you go. Keep at it, and your skills will grow over time.

Try Other Strategies

In addition to being prepared with your "no thanks," consider these strategies:

- Have nonalcoholic drinks always in hand if you are quitting, or as "drink spacers" between drinks if you are cutting back.
- Keep track of every drink if you are cutting back so you stay within your limits.
- Ask for support from others to cope with temptation.
- Plan an escape if the temptation gets too great.
- Ask others to refrain from pressuring you or drinking in your presence (this can be hard).

If you have successfully refused drink offers before, then recall what worked and build on it.

REMEMBER, IT IS YOUR CHOICE

How you think about any decision to change can affect your success. Many people who decide to cut back or quit drinking think, "I am not allowed to drink," as if an external authority were imposing rules on them. Thoughts like this can breed resentment and make it easier to give in. It is important to challenge this kind of thinking by telling yourself that you are in charge, that you know how you want your life to be, and that you have decided to make a change.

Similarly, you may worry about how others will react or view you if you make a change. Again, challenge these thoughts by remembering that it is your life and your choice, and that your decision should be respected.

PLAN AHEAD TO STAY IN CONTROL

As you change your drinking, it is normal and common to have urges or a craving for alcohol. The words "urge" and "craving" refer to a broad range of thoughts, physical sensations, or emotions that tempt you to drink, even though you have at least some desire not to. You may feel an uncomfortable pull in two directions or sense a loss of control.

Fortunately, urges to drink are short-lived, predictable, and controllable. With time, and by practicing new responses, you will find that your urges to drink will lose strength, and you will gain confidence in your ability to deal with urges that may still arise at times. If you are having a very difficult time with urges, or do not make progress with the strategies after a few weeks, then consult a doctor or therapist for support. In addition, some new, nonhabit forming medications can reduce the desire to drink or lessen the rewarding effect of drinking so it is easier to stop.

RECOGNIZE TWO TYPES OF TRIGGERS

An urge to drink can be set off by external triggers in the environment and internal ones within yourself.

- **External triggers** are people, places, things, or times of day that offer drinking opportunities or remind you of drinking. These "high-risk situations" are more obvious, predictable, and avoidable than internal triggers.
- **Internal triggers** can be puzzling because the urge to drink just seems to "pop up." But, if you pause to think about it when it happens, you will find that the urge may have been set off by a fleeting thought, a positive emotion such as excitement, a negative emotion, such as frustration, or a physical sensation such as a headache, tension, or nervousness.

Consider tracking and analyzing your urges to drink for a couple of weeks. This will help you become more aware of when and how you experience urges, what triggers them, and ways to avoid or control them.

AVOID HIGH-RISK SITUATIONS

In many cases, your best strategy will be to avoid taking the chance that you will have an urge, then slip and drink. At home, keep little or no alcohol. Socially, avoid activities involving drinking. If you feel guilty about turning down an invitation, remind yourself that you are not necessarily talking about "forever." When the urges subside or become more manageable, you may decide to ease gradually into some situations you now choose to avoid. In the meantime, you can stay connected with friends by suggesting alternate activities that do not involve drinking.

COPE WITH TRIGGERS YOU CANNOT AVOID

It is not possible to avoid all high-risk situations or to block internal triggers, so you will need a range of strategies to handle urges to drink. Here are some options:

- **Remind yourself** of your reasons for making a change. Carry your top reasons on a wallet card or in an electronic message that you can access easily, such as a mobile phone notepad entry or a saved e-mail.
- **Talk it through** with someone you trust. Have a trusted friend on standby for a phone call, or bring one along to high-risk situations.
- **Distract yourself** with a healthy, alternative activity. For different situations, come up with engaging short, mid-range, and longer options, like texting or calling someone, watching short online videos, lifting weights to music, showering, meditating, taking a walk, or doing a hobby.
- **Challenge the thought** that drives the urge. Stop it, analyze the error in it, and replace it.

Example: "It could not hurt to have one little drink. WAIT a minute—what am I thinking? One could hurt, as I have seen 'just one' lead to lots more. I am sticking with my choice not to drink."

- **Ride it out** without giving in. Instead of fighting an urge, accept it as normal and temporary. As you ride it out, keep in mind that it will soon crest like an ocean wave and pass.
- **Leave** high-risk situations quickly and gracefully. It helps to plan your escape in advance.

Chapter 40 | **Coping with Stress**

Chapter Contents

Section 40.1 | How to Cope with Your Stress

This section includes text excerpted from "Coping with Stress," Centers for Disease Control and Prevention (CDC), September 3, 2019.

Everyone—adults, teens, and even children, experiences stress. Stress is a reaction to a situation where a person feels threatened or anxious. Stress can be positive (e.g., preparing for a wedding) or negative (e.g., dealing with a natural disaster). Learning healthy ways to cope and getting the right care and support can help reduce stressful feelings and symptoms.

After a traumatic event, people may have strong and lingering reactions. These events may include personal or environmental disasters or threats with an assault. The symptoms may be physical or emotional. Common reactions to a stressful event can include:
- Disbelief, shock, and numbness
- Feeling sad, frustrated, and helpless
- Difficulty concentrating and making decisions
- Headaches, back pains, and stomach problems
- Smoking or use of alcohol or drugs

HEALTHY WAYS TO COPE WITH STRESS

Feeling emotional and nervous or having trouble sleeping and eating can all be normal reactions to stress. Here are some healthy ways you can deal with stress:
- **Take care of yourself.**
  - Eat healthy, well-balanced meals
  - Exercise on a regular basis
  - Get plenty of sleep
  - Give yourself a break if you feel stressed out
- **Talk to others**. Share your problems and how you are feeling and coping with a parent, friend, counselor, doctor, or pastor.
- **Avoid drugs and alcohol.** These may seem to help, but they can create additional problems and increase the stress you are already feeling.

- **Take a break**. If news events are causing your stress, take a break from listening or watching the news.
- **Recognize when you need more help**. If problems continue or you are thinking about suicide, talk to a psychologist, social worker, or professional counselor.

HELPING YOUTH COPE WITH STRESS

Children and adolescents often struggle with how to cope with stress. Youth can be particularly overwhelmed when their stress is connected to a traumatic event—such as a natural disaster, family loss, school shootings, or community violence. Parents and educators can take steps to provide stability and support that help young people feel better.

Tips for Parents

It is natural for children to worry when scary or stressful events happen in their lives. Talking to your children about these events can help put frightening information into a more balanced setting. Monitor what children see and hear about stressful events happening in their lives. Here are some suggestions to help children cope:

- **Maintain a normal routine.** Helping children wake up, go to sleep, and eat meals at regular times provide them a sense of stability. Going to school and participating in typical after-school activities also provide stability and extra support.
- **Talk, listen, and encourage expression.** Create opportunities for your children to talk, but do not force them. Listen to your child's thoughts and feelings and share some of yours. After a traumatic event, it is important for children to feel they can share their feelings and that you understand their fears and worries. Keep having these conversations. Ask them regularly how they feel in a week, in a month, and so on.
- **Watch and listen.** Be alert for any change in behavior. Are children sleeping more or less? Are they

withdrawing from friends or family? Any changes in behavior may be signs that your child is having trouble and may need support.

- **Reassure.** Stressful events can challenge a child's sense of safety and security. Reassure your child about her or his safety and well-being. Discuss ways that you, the school, and the community are taking steps to keep them safe.
- **Connect with others.** Talk to other parents and your child's teachers about ways to help your child cope. It is often helpful for parents, schools, and health professionals to work together for the well-being of all children in stressful times.

Tips for Kids and Teens

After a traumatic event, it is normal to feel anxious about your safety and security. Even if you were not directly involved, you may worry about whether this type of event may someday affect you. Check out the tips below for some ideas to help deal with these fears.

- **Talk to and stay connected to others.** This might be:
  - Parents, or other relatives
  - Friends
  - Teachers
  - Coach
  - Family doctor
  - Member of your place of worship

  Talking with someone can help you make sense out of your experience and figure out ways to feel better. If you are not sure where to turn, call your local crisis intervention center or a national hotline.
- **Get active.** Go for a walk, play sports, play a musical instrument, or join an after-school program. Volunteer with a community group that promotes nonviolence or another school or community activity that you care about. These can be positive ways to handle your feelings and to see that things are going to get better.

- **Take care of yourself.** Try to get plenty of sleep, eat right, exercise, and keep a normal routine. By keeping yourself healthy, you will be better able to handle a tough time.
- **Take information breaks.** Pictures and stories about a disaster can increase worry and other stressful feelings. Taking breaks from the news, Internet, and conversations about the disaster can help calm you down.

Tips for School Personnel

School personnel can help their students restore their sense of safety by talking with the children about their fears. Other tips for school personnel include:

- **Reach out and talk.** Create opportunities to have students talk, but do not force them. Try asking questions like, what do you think about these events, or how do you think these things happen? You can be a model by sharing some of your own thoughts as well as correct misinformation. When children talk about their feelings, it can help them cope and to know that different feelings are normal.
- **Watch and listen.** Be alert for any change in behavior. Are students withdrawing from friends? Acting out? These changes may be early signs that a student is struggling and needs extra support from the school and family.
- **Maintain normal routines.** A regular classroom and school schedule can provide a sense of stability and safety. Encourage students to keep up with their schoolwork and extracurricular activities but do not push them if they seem overwhelmed.
- **Take care of yourself.** You are better able to support your students if you are healthy, coping and taking care of yourself first.
  - Eat healthy, well-balanced meals.
  - Exercise on a regular basis.

- Get plenty of sleep.
- Give yourself a break if you feel stressed out.

Section 40.2 | Benefits of Support Animals

This section includes text excerpted from "The Power of Pets—Health Benefits of Human-Animal Interactions," *NIH News in Health*, National Institutes of Health (NIH), February 2018; Text under the heading "Service Animals for Mental-Health Concerns" is © 2020 Omnigraphics. Reviewed August 2020.

Nothing compares to the joy of coming home to a loyal companion. The unconditional love of a pet can do more than keep you company. Pets may also decrease stress, improve heart health, and even help children with their emotional and social skills.

An estimated 68 percent of the U.S. households have a pet. But, who benefits from an animal? And which type of pet brings health benefits?

Over the past 10 years, the National Institutes of Health (NIH) has partnered with the Mars Corporation's WALTHAM Centre for Pet Nutrition to answer questions such as these by funding research studies.

Scientists are looking at what the potential physical and mental-health benefits are for different animals—from fish to guinea pigs to dogs and cats.

POSSIBLE HEALTH EFFECTS

Research on human-animal interactions is still relatively new. Some studies have shown positive health effects, but the results have been mixed.

Interacting with animals has been shown to decrease levels of cortisol (a stress-related hormone) and lower blood pressure. Other studies have found that animals can reduce loneliness, increase feelings of social support, and boost your mood.

The NIH/Mars Partnership is funding a range of studies focused on the relationships we have with animals. For example, researchers are looking into how animals might influence child development. They are studying animal interactions with kids who have autism, attention deficit hyperactivity disorder (ADHD), and other conditions.

"There is not one answer about how a pet can help somebody with a specific condition," explains Dr. Layla Esposito, who oversees NIH's Human-Animal Interaction (HAI) Research Program. "Is your goal to increase physical activity? Then you might benefit from owning a dog. You have to walk a dog several times a day and you are going to increase physical activity. If your goal is reducing stress, sometimes watching fish swim can result in a feeling of calmness. So there is no one-size-fits-all."

The NIH is funding large-scale surveys to find out the range of pets people live with and how their relationships with their pets relate to health.

"We are trying to tap into the subjective quality of the relationship with the animal—that part of the bond that people feel with animals—and how that translates into some of the health benefits," explains Dr. James Griffin, a child development expert at NIH.

ANIMALS HELPING PEOPLE
Animals can serve as a source of comfort and support. Therapy dogs are especially good at this. They are sometimes brought into hospitals or nursing homes to help reduce patients' stress and anxiety.

"Dogs are very present. If someone is struggling with something, they know how to sit there and be loving," says Dr. Ann Berger, a physician, and researcher at the NIH Clinical Center (CC) in Bethesda, Maryland. "Their attention is focused on the person all the time."

Berger works with people who have cancer and terminal illnesses. She teaches them about mindfulness to help decrease stress and manage pain.

"The foundations of mindfulness include attention, intention, compassion, and awareness," Berger says. "All of those things are things that animals bring to the table. People kind of have to learn it. Animals do this innately."

Researchers are studying the safety of bringing animals into hospital settings because animals may expose people to more germs.

A current study is looking at the safety of bringing dogs to visit children with cancer, Esposito says. Scientists will be testing the children's hands to see if there are dangerous levels of germs transferred from the dog after the visit.

Dogs may also aid in the classroom. One study found that dogs can help children with ADHD focus their attention. Researchers enrolled two groups of children diagnosed with ADHD in 12-week group therapy sessions. The first group of kids read to a therapy dog once a week for 30 minutes. The second group read to puppets that looked like dogs.

Kids who read to the real animals showed better social skills and more sharing, cooperation, and volunteering. They also had fewer behavioral problems.

Another study found that children with autism spectrum disorder were calmer while playing with guinea pigs in the classroom. When the children spent 10 minutes in a supervised group playtime with guinea pigs, their anxiety levels dropped. The children also had better social interactions and were more engaged with their peers. The researchers suggest that the animals offered unconditional acceptance, making them a calm comfort to the children.

"Animals can become a way of building a bridge for those social interactions," Griffin says. He adds that researchers are trying to better understand these effects and who they might help.

Animals may help you in other unexpected ways. A study showed that caring for fish helped teens with diabetes better manage their disease. Researchers had a group of teens with type 1 diabetes care for a pet fish twice a day by feeding and checking water levels. The caretaking routine also included changing the tank water each week. This was paired with the children reviewing their blood glucose (blood sugar) logs with parents.

Researchers tracked how consistently these teens checked their blood glucose. Compared with teens who were not given a fish to care for, fish-keeping teens were more disciplined about checking their own blood glucose levels, which is essential for maintaining their health.

While pets may bring a wide range of health benefits, an animal may not work for everyone. Studies suggest that early exposure to pets may help protect young children from developing allergies and asthma. But, for people who are allergic to certain animals, having pets in the home can do more harm than good.

HELPING EACH OTHER

Pets also bring new responsibilities. Knowing how to care for and feed an animal is part of owning a pet. NIH/Mars funds study looking into the effects of human-animal interactions for both the pet and the person.

Remember that animals can feel stressed and fatigued, too. It is important for kids to be able to recognize signs of stress in their pets and know when not to approach. Animal bites can cause serious harm.

"Dog bite prevention is certainly an issue parents need to consider, especially for young children who do not always know the boundaries of what is appropriate to do with a dog," Esposito explains.

SERVICE ANIMALS FOR MENTAL-HEALTH CONCERNS

Service animals are usually trained to help people with disabilities such as blindness. However, they can also be of help to individuals with medical conditions and psychiatric problems. There are two types of service or support animals for people with mental-health concerns: psychiatric service animals and emotional support animals. However, both these animals are designated for serving very different purposes and people can train these animals to do specific tasks according to their individual needs.

Psychiatric Service Animals

A person diagnosed with a psychiatric disorder that impairs their daily functioning can be assigned a psychiatric service animal to support them with their daily activities. These animals are recognized by the Americans with Disabilities Act (ADA). Psychiatric service animals such as specially trained dogs assist people with severe anxiety, depression, and posttraumatic stress disorder (PTSD). These dogs can help accompany their owners to public places and lead them to safe place if they sense or predict any panic attack. They are also trained to prevent impulsive or destructive behaviors, such as self-harm or self-mutilation.

Emotional Support Animals

People with a social anxiety disorder (SAD) often derive a sense of comfort from the presence of an animal. An emotional support animal is a dog or other such domesticated animal that gives therapeutic support to the elderly as well as people with no severe mental-health concerns. These animals are not specially trained, and the ADA does not grant them the same rights to access public spaces. Many other federal laws that cover psychiatric service animals do not apply to emotional service animals.

References

1. Duffly, Zachary. "Psychiatric Service Dogs & Emotional Support Animals: Access to Public Places & Other Settings," Nolo, October 19, 2012.
2. Cuncic, Arlin. "How Psychiatric Service Animals Help Social Anxiety Disorder," Very Well Mind, July 22, 2019.

Chapter 41 | Managing Anxiety and Stress Related to COVID-19

On February 11, 2020, the World Health Organization (WHO) announced an official name for the disease that is causing the 2019 novel coronavirus outbreak, first identified in Wuhan China. The new name of this disease is coronavirus disease 2019, abbreviated as COVID-19.

The COVID-19 pandemic may be stressful for people. Fear and anxiety about a new disease and what could happen can be overwhelming and cause strong emotions in adults and children. Public-health actions, such as social distancing, can make people feel isolated and lonely and can increase stress and anxiety. However, these actions are necessary to reduce the spread of COVID-19. Coping with stress in a healthy way will make you, the people you care about, and your community stronger.

EVERYONE REACTS DIFFERENTLY TO STRESSFUL SITUATIONS

How you respond to stress during the COVID-19 pandemic can depend on your background, your social support from family or friends, your financial situation, your health and emotional background, the community you live in, and many other factors. The changes that can happen because of the COVID-19 pandemic and the ways we try to contain the spread of the virus can affect anyone.

This chapter includes text excerpted from "Coping with Stress," Centers for Disease Control and Prevention (CDC), July 1, 2020.

People who may respond more strongly to the stress of a crisis include:

- People who are at higher risk for severe illness from COVID-19 (e.g., older people, and people of any age with certain underlying medical conditions)
- Children and teens
- People caring for family members or loved ones
- Frontline workers, such as healthcare providers and first responders
- Essential workers who work in the food industry
- People who have existing mental-health conditions
- People who use substances or have a substance-use disorder (SUD)
- People who have lost their jobs, had their work hours reduced, or had other major changes to their employment
- People who have disabilities or developmental delay
- People who are socially isolated from others, including people who live alone, and people in rural or frontier areas
- People in some racial and ethnic minority groups
- People who do not have access to information in their primary language
- People experiencing homelessness
- People who live in congregate (group) settings

RECOVERING FROM COVID-19 OR ENDING HOME ISOLATION

It can be stressful to be separated from others if you have or were exposed to COVID-19. Each person ending a period of home isolation may feel differently about it.

Emotional reactions may include:

- Mixed emotions, including relief
- Fear and worry about your own health and the health of your loved ones
- Stress from the experience of having COVID-19 and monitoring yourself, or being monitored by others

- Sadness, anger, or frustration because friends or loved ones have fears of getting the disease from you, even though you are cleared to be around others
- Guilt about not being able to perform normal work or parenting duties while you had COVID-19
- Worry about getting reinfected or sick again even though you have already had COVID-19
- Other emotional or mental-health changes

Children may also feel upset or have other strong emotions if they, or someone they know, has COVID-19, even if they are now better and able to be around others again.

TAKE CARE OF YOURSELF AND YOUR COMMUNITY

Taking care of your friends and your family can be a stress reliever, but it should be balanced with care for yourself. Helping others cope with their stress such as by providing social support, can also make your community stronger. During times of increased social distancing, people can still maintain social connections and care for their mental health. Phone calls or video chats can help you and your loved ones feel socially connected, less lonely, or isolated.

Healthy Ways to Cope with Stress

- Know what to do if you are sick and are concerned about COVID-19. Contact a health professional before you start any self-treatment for COVID-19.
- Know where and how to get treatment and other support services and resources, including counseling or therapy (in person or through telehealth services).
- Take care of your emotional health. Taking care of your emotional health will help you think clearly and react to the urgent needs to protect yourself and your family.
- Take breaks from watching, reading, or listening to news stories, including those on social media. Hearing about the pandemic repeatedly can be upsetting.
  - Take care of your body.

- Take deep breaths, stretch, or meditate.
- Try to eat healthy, well-balanced meals.
- Exercise regularly.
- Get plenty of sleep.
- Avoid excessive alcohol and drug use.
- Make time to unwind. Try to do some other activities you enjoy.
- Connect with others. Talk with people you trust about your concerns and how you are feeling.
- Connect with your community- or faith-based organizations. While social distancing measures are in place, consider connecting online, through social media, or by phone or e-mail.

Know the Facts to Help Reduce Stress

Knowing the facts about COVID-19 and stopping the spread of rumors can help reduce stress and stigma. Understanding the risk to yourself and people you care about can help you connect with others and make an outbreak less stressful.

TAKE CARE OF YOUR MENTAL HEALTH

Mental health is an important part of overall health and well-being. It affects how we think, feel, and act. It may also affect how we handle stress, relate to others, and make choices during an emergency.

People with preexisting mental-health conditions or SUD may be particularly vulnerable in an emergency. Mental-health conditions (such as depression, anxiety, bipolar disorder, or schizophrenia) affect a person's thinking, feeling, mood, or behavior in a way that influences their ability to relate to others and function each day. These conditions may be situational (short term) or long-lasting (chronic). People with preexisting mental-health conditions should continue with their treatment and be aware of new or worsening symptoms. If you think you have new or worse symptoms, call your healthcare provider.

Call your healthcare provider if stress gets in the way of your daily activities for several days in a row. Free and confidential resources can also help you or a loved one connect with a skilled, trained counselor in your area.

Get Immediate Help in a Crisis

- Call 911
- Disaster Distress Helpline: 800-985-5990 (press 2 for Spanish), or text TalkWithUs for English or Hablanos for Spanish to 66746. Spanish speakers from Puerto Rico can text Hablanos to 787-339-2663.
- National Suicide Prevention Lifeline (NSPL): 800-273-TALK (800-273-8255) for English, 888-628-9454 for Spanish, or Lifeline Crisis Chat
- National Domestic Violence Hotline: 800-799-7233 or text LOVEIS to 22522
- National Child Abuse Hotline: 800-4AChild (800-422-4453) or text 800-422-4453
- National Sexual Assault Hotline: 800-656-HOPE (800-656-4673) or Online Chat
- The Eldercare Locator: 800-677-1116 TTY Instructions
- Veteran's Crisis Line: 800-273-TALK (800-273-8255) or Crisis Chat or text: 8388255

Find a Healthcare Provider or Treatment for Substance-Use Disorder and Mental Health

- Substance Abuse and Mental Health Services Administration's (SAMHSA) National Helpline: 800-662-HELP (800-662-4357) and TTY 800-487-4889
- Treatment Services Locator Website (findtreatment. samhsa.gov/)
- Interactive Map of Selected Federally Qualified Health Centers (FQHCs)

Suicide

Different life experiences affect a person's risk for suicide. For example, suicide risk is higher among people who have experienced violence, including child abuse, bullying, or sexual violence.

Feelings of isolation, depression, anxiety, and other emotional or financial stresses are known to raise the risk for suicide. People may be more likely to experience these feelings during a crisis like a pandemic.

However, there are ways to protect against suicidal thoughts and behaviors. For example, support from family and community, or feeling connected, and having access to in-person or virtual counseling or therapy can help with suicidal thoughts and behavior, particularly during a crisis like the COVID-19 pandemic.

Part 6 | Looking Ahead

Chapter 42 | **Guiding Principles of Recovery**

Recovery is a process of change through which people improve their health and wellness, live self-directed lives, and strive to reach their full potential. There are four major dimensions that support recovery:

- **Health**—overcoming or managing one's disease(s) or symptoms and making informed, healthy choices that support physical and emotional well-being.
- **Home**—having a stable and safe place to live.
- **Purpose**—conducting meaningful daily activities and having the independence, income, and resources to participate in society
- **Community**—having relationships and social networks that provide support, friendship, love, and hope.

Hope, the belief that these challenges and conditions can be overcome, is the foundation of recovery. The process of recovery is highly personal and occurs via many pathways. Recovery is characterized by continual growth and improvement in one's health and wellness that may involve setbacks. Because setbacks are a natural part of life, resilience becomes a key component of recovery.

The process of recovery is supported through relationships and social networks. This often involves family members who become

This chapter contains text excerpted from the following sources: Text in this chapter begins with excerpts from "Recovery and Recovery Support," Substance Abuse and Mental Health Services Administration (SAMHSA), April 23, 2020; Text beginning with the heading "Recovery Emerges from Hope" is excerpted from "SAMHSA's Working Definition of Recovery," Substance Abuse and Mental Health Services Administration (SAMHSA), 2012. Reviewed August 2020.

the champions of their loved one's recovery. Families of people in recovery may experience adversities that lead to increased family stress, guilt, shame, anger, fear, anxiety, loss, grief, and isolation. The concept of resilience in recovery is also vital for family members who need access to intentional supports that promote their health and well-being. The support of peers and friends is also crucial in engaging and supporting individuals in recovery.

Recovery services and supports must be flexible. What may work for adults may be very different for youth or older adults. For example, the nature of social supports, peer mentors, and recovery coaching for adolescents is different than for adults and older adults. Supporting recovery requires that mental health and addiction services:

- Be responsive and respectful to the health beliefs, practices, and cultural and linguistic needs of diverse people and groups.
- Actively address diversity in the delivery of services.
- Seek to reduce health disparities in access and outcomes.

RECOVERY EMERGES FROM HOPE

The belief that recovery is real provides the essential and motivating message of a better future—that people can and do overcome the internal and external challenges, barriers, and obstacles that confront them. Hope is internalized and can be fostered by peers, families, providers, allies, and others. Hope is the catalyst of the recovery process.

RECOVERY IS PERSON-DRIVEN

Self-determination and self-direction are the foundations for recovery as individuals define their own life goals and design their unique path(s) towards those goals. Individuals optimize their autonomy and independence to the greatest extent possible by leading, controlling, and exercising choice over the services and supports that assist their recovery and resilience. In doing so, they are empowered and provided with the resources to make informed decisions, initiate recovery, build on their strengths, and gain or regain control over their lives.

RECOVERY OCCURS VIA MANY PATHWAYS

Individuals are unique with distinct needs, strengths, preferences, goals, culture, and backgrounds—including trauma experience—that affect and determine their pathway(s) to recovery. Recovery is built on the multiple capacities, strengths, talents, coping abilities, resources, and inherent value of each individual. Recovery pathways are highly personalized. They may include professional clinical treatment; use of medications; support from families and in schools; faith-based approaches; peer support; and other approaches. Recovery is nonlinear, characterized by continual growth and improved functioning that may involve setbacks. Because setbacks are a natural, though not inevitable, part of the recovery process, it is essential to foster resilience for all individuals and families. Abstinence from the use of alcohol, illicit drugs, and nonprescribed medications is the goal for those with addictions. The use of tobacco and nonprescribed or illicit drugs is not safe for anyone. In some cases, recovery pathways can be enabled by creating a supportive environment. This is especially true for children, who may not have the legal or developmental capacity to set their own course.

RECOVERY IS HOLISTIC

Recovery encompasses an individual's whole life, including mind, body, spirit, and community. This includes addressing: self-care practices, family, housing, employment, transportation, education, clinical treatment for mental disorders and substance-use disorders (SUD), services and supports, primary healthcare, dental care, complementary and alternative services, faith, spirituality, creativity, social networks, and community participation. The array of services and supports available should be integrated and coordinated.

RECOVERY IS SUPPORTED BY PEERS AND ALLIES

Mutual support and mutual aid groups, including the sharing of experiential knowledge and skills, as well as social learning, play an invaluable role in recovery. Peers encourage and engage other peers and provide each other with a vital sense of belonging, supportive relationships, valued roles, and community. Through helping others and giving back to the community, one helps one's self. Peer-operated supports and services provide important resources to assist people along their journeys of recovery and wellness. Professionals can also play an important role in the recovery process by providing clinical treatment and other services that support individuals in their chosen recovery paths. While peers and allies play an important role for many in recovery, their role for children and youth may be slightly different. Peer supports for families are very important for children with behavioral-health problems and can also play a supportive role for youth in recovery.

RECOVERY IS SUPPORTED THROUGH RELATIONSHIP AND SOCIAL NETWORKS

An important factor in the recovery process is the presence and involvement of people who believe in the person's ability to recover; who offer hope, support, and encouragement; and who also suggest strategies and resources for change. Family members, peers, providers, faith groups, community members, and other allies form vital support networks. Through these relationships, people leave unhealthy and/or unfulfilling life roles behind and engage in new roles (e.g., partner, caregiver, friend, student, employee) that lead to a greater sense of belonging, personhood, empowerment, autonomy, social inclusion, and community participation.

RECOVERY IS CULTURALLY-BASED AND INFLUENCED

Culture and cultural background in all of its diverse representations— including values, traditions, and beliefs—are keys in determining a person's journey and unique pathway to recovery. Services should be culturally grounded, attuned, sensitive, congruent, and competent, as well as personalized to meet each individual's unique needs.

RECOVERY IS SUPPORTED BY ADDRESSING TRAUMA

The experience of trauma (such as physical or sexual abuse, domestic violence, war, disaster, and others) is often a precursor to or associated with alcohol and drug use, mental-health problems, and related issues. Services and supports should be trauma-informed to foster safety (physical and emotional) and trust, as well as promote choice, empowerment, and collaboration.

RECOVERY INVOLVES INDIVIDUAL, FAMILY, AND COMMUNITY STRENGTHS AND RESPONSIBILITY

Individuals, families, and communities have strengths and resources that serve as a foundation for recovery. In addition, individuals have a personal responsibility for their own self-care and journeys of recovery. Individuals should be supported in speaking for themselves. Families and significant others have responsibilities to support their loved ones, especially for children and youth in recovery. Communities have responsibilities to provide opportunities and resources to address discrimination and to foster social inclusion and recovery. Individuals in recovery also have a social responsibility and should have the ability to join with peers to speak collectively about their strengths, needs, wants, desires, and aspirations.

RECOVERY IS BASED ON RESPECT

Community, systems, and societal acceptance and appreciation for people affected by mental-health and substance-use problems—including protecting their rights and eliminating discrimination—are crucial in achieving recovery. There is a need to acknowledge that taking steps towards recovery may require great courage. Self-acceptance, developing a positive and meaningful sense of identity, and regaining belief in one's self are particularly important.

Chapter 43 | Family: An Important Social Context for Recovery

When someone is affected by mental illness or addiction, it can affect the entire family. When that person enters treatment, the family's pain and confusion do not just go away. How does any family member move past the damage that has occurred? How does the family as a whole strengthen the ties that hold it together?

Family therapy is one answer. It works together with individual therapy for the benefit of all family members.

WHAT IS FAMILY THERAPY?

Family therapy is based on the idea that a family is a system of different parts. A change in any part of the system will trigger changes in all the other parts. This means that when one member of a family is affected by a behavioral-health disorder, such as mental illness or addiction, everyone is affected.

As a result, family dynamics can change in unhealthy ways. Lies and secrets can build up in the family. Some family members may take on too much responsibility, other family members may act out, and some may just shut down.

Sometimes conditions at home are already unhappy before a family member's mental illness or addiction emerges. That person's changing behaviors can throw the family into even greater turmoil.

This chapter includes text excerpted from "Family Therapy Can Help," Substance Abuse and Mental Health Services Administration (SAMHSA), 2013. Reviewed August 2020.

Often a family remains stuck in unhealthy patterns even after the family member with the behavioral-health disorder moves into recovery. Even in the best circumstances, families can find it hard to adjust to the person in their midst who is recovering, who is behaving differently than before, and who needs support.

Family therapy can help the family as a whole recover and heal. It can help all members of the family make specific, positive changes as the person in recovery changes. These changes can help all family members heal from the trauma of mental illness or addiction.

WHO CAN ATTEND FAMILY THERAPY?

"Family" means a group of two or more people with close and enduring emotional ties. Using this definition, each person in treatment for a behavioral-health disorder has a unique set of family members. Therapists do not decide who should be in family therapy. Instead they ask, "Who is most important to you?"

- Parents
- Spouses or partners
- In-laws
- Siblings
- Children
- Elected, chosen, or honorary
- Family members
- Other relatives
- Stepparents
- Stepchildren
- Foster parents
- Foster children
- Godparents
- Godchildren
- Blended family members
- Extended family members
- Friends
- Fellow Veterans
- Colleagues who care
- Mentors
- Mutual-help group members
- Sponsors

Sometimes members of a family live together, but sometimes they live apart. Either way, if they are considered family by the person in treatment, they can be included in family therapy.

WHEN SHOULD FAMILY THERAPY START?

Family therapy is typically introduced after the individual in treatment for mental illness or addiction has made progress in recovery. This could be a few months after treatment starts, or a year or more later.

Timing is important because people new to recovery have a lot to do. They are working to remain stable in their new patterns of behavior and ways of thinking. They are just beginning to face the many changes they must make to stay mentally healthy or to remain sober. They are learning such things as how to deal with urges to fall into old patterns, how to resist triggers and cravings, how to adhere to medication regimens, and how to avoid temptations to rationalize and make excuses. For them to explore family issues at the same time can be too much. It can potentially contribute to relapse into mental illness or substance using behaviors.

Family therapy tends to be most helpful once the person in treatment is fully committed to the recovery process and is ready to make more changes. The person's counselor can advise on the best time to start family therapy.

WHAT ARE THE GOALS OF FAMILY THERAPY?

There are two main goals in family therapy. One goal is to help everyone give the right kind of support to the family member in behavioral-health treatment, so that recovery sticks and relapse is avoided. The other goal is to strengthen the whole family's emotional health, so that everyone can thrive.

Specific objectives for family therapy are unique to each family, and these objectives may change over time. The family decides for itself what to focus on, and when.

HOW IS FAMILY THERAPY ORGANIZED?

Family therapy involves the entire family meeting together. Sometimes part of the family meets. The family therapist may work one-on-one with a particular family member, in addition to the family sessions, although this is not typical.

WHAT HAPPENS IN A PARTICULAR SESSION

There are many things that can happen in family therapy. A session can be devoted to talking about family concerns and how people are feeling. Family members might use the session to talk about a particular crisis or problem that needs solving. Or, they might want to focus on the changes that have been happening.

Another possible topic for a family therapy session is coping skills such as how to deal with anger, regret, or sadness. Sometimes just letting out feelings and talking about them in therapy sessions can bring relief, understanding, and healing.

The focus of a session might be on learning how to communicate more effectively with each other. For example, the therapist might coach a family member to speak up, to practice saying "no" to unreasonable demands, or to give a compliment. Family members might be asked to rephrase a statement in a more positive way. The therapist also might help family members improve their listening and observing skills to reduce misunderstanding.

Sometimes the therapist asks family members to do homework before the next session. For example, the therapist might ask family members to watch for nice things that other family members say during the week. The therapist might ask family members to eat a meal together or to do something fun together, like play board games or go bowling. The homework is designed to help family members practice new and healthier ways of behaving with each other.

IS FAMILY THERAPY EFFECTIVE?

Research suggests that behavioral-health treatment that includes family therapy works better than treatment that does not. For people with mental illness, family therapy in conjunction with individual treatment can increase medication adherence, reduce rates of relapse and rehospitalization, reduce psychiatric symptoms, and relieve stress.

Family: An Important Social Context for Recovery

For people with addiction, family therapy can help them decide to enter or stay in treatment. It can reduce their risk of dropping out of treatment. It also can reduce their continued use of alcohol or drugs, discourage relapse, and promote long-term recovery.

Family therapy benefits other family members besides the person in treatment. By making positive changes in family dynamics, the therapy can reduce the burden of stress that other family members feel. It can prevent additional family members from moving into drug or alcohol use. Research also shows that family therapy can improve how couples treat each other, how children behave, how the whole family gets along, and how the family connects with its neighbors.

Family therapy is not always easy. There will be struggles for everyone involved, but the outcome is worth it. Family therapy is an effective way to help the person in treatment, while also helping the family as a whole.

Chapter 44 | Importance of Peer Support in Recovery

WHAT IS PEER SUPPORT?

Peer support encompasses a range of activities and interactions between people who have shared similar experiences of being diagnosed with mental-health conditions. This mutuality—often called "peerness"—between a peer worker and person using services promotes connection and inspires hope.

Peer support offers a level of acceptance, understanding, and validation not found in many other professional relationships. "I am an expert at not being an expert, and that takes a lot of expertise," said one (anonymous) peer worker, highlighting the supportive rather than directive nature of the peer relationship. By sharing their own lived experience and practical guidance, peer workers help people to develop their own goals, create strategies for self-empowerment, and take concrete steps towards building fulfilling, self-determined lives for themselves.

WHAT DO PEER SUPPORT SPECIALISTS DO?
Support the Recovery of Individuals

Peer workers offer encouragement, practical assistance, guidance, and understanding to support recovery. Peer support workers walk alongside people in recovery, offering individualized supports and demonstrating that recovery is possible. They share their own lived

This chapter includes text excerpted from "Peers Supporting Recovery from Mental Health Conditions," Substance Abuse and Mental Health Services Administration (SAMHSA), November 26, 2017.

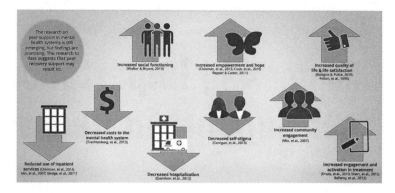

Figure 44.1. Is Peer Recovery Support Effective for People with Mental-Health Conditions?

experience of moving from hopelessness to hope. They share tools that can complement or replace clinical supports by providing strategies for self-empowerment and achieving a self-determined life. They support people in recovery to connect with their own inner strength, motivation, and desire to move forward in life, even when experiencing challenges. Peer workers offer different types of support, including:

- Emotional (empathy and camaraderie)
- Informational (connections to information and referrals to community resources that support health and wellness)
- Instrumental (concrete supports such as housing or employment)
- Affiliational support (connections to community supports, activities, and events)

Improve Mental-Health Systems

Peer support is valuable not only for the person receiving services, but also for behavioral-health professionals and the systems in which they work. Peer workers educate their colleagues and advance the field by sharing their perspectives and experience in order to increase understanding of how practices and policies may be improved to promote wellness and resiliency. This is particularly important in mental-health systems, where historical oppression, violence, and discrimination present significant barriers to recovery for many people. Peer workers play vital roles in moving behavioral-health professionals and systems towards recovery orientation.

Chapter 45 | Building Psychological Resilience

Chapter Contents

Section 45.1 | Positive Mental Health and Resilience

This section includes text excerpted from "Individual Resilience," Office of the Assistant Secretary for Preparedness and Response (ASPR), U.S. Department of Health and Human Services (HHS), January 29, 2018.

WHAT IS INDIVIDUAL RESILIENCE?

Individual resilience involves behaviors, thoughts, and actions that promote personal well-being and mental health. People can develop the ability to withstand, adapt to, and recover from stress and adversity—and maintain or return to a state of mental health well-being—by using effective coping strategies. This is called "individual resilience."

A disaster can impair resilience due to stress, traumatic exposure, distressing psychological reactions, and disrupted social networks. Feelings of grief, sadness, and a range of other emotions are common after traumatic events. Resilient individuals, however, are able to work through the emotions and effects of stress and painful events and rebuild their lives.

WHAT CONTRIBUTES TO INDIVIDUAL RESILIENCE

People develop resilience by learning better skills and strategies for managing stress and better ways of thinking about life's challenges. To be resilient one must tap into personal strengths and the support of family, friends, neighbors, and/or faith communities.

WHAT ARE THE CHARACTERISTICS THAT SUPPORT INDIVIDUAL RESILIENCE?

Age, gender, health, biology, education level, cultural beliefs and traditions, and economic resources can play important roles in psychological resilience. The following characteristics also contribute to individual resilience:

- **Social support and close relationships with family and friends.** People who have close social support and strong connections with family and friends are able to get help during tough times and also enjoy their relationships during everyday life.

333

- **The ability to manage strong feelings and impulses.** People who are able to manage strong emotions are less likely to get overwhelmed, frustrated, or aggressive. People who are able to manage feelings can still feel sadness or loss, but they are also able to find healthy ways to cope and heal.
- **Good problem-solving skills.** People problem-solve daily. Thinking, planning, and solving problems in an organized way are important skills. Problem-solving skills contribute to feelings of independence and self-competence.
- **Feeling in control.** After the chaos of a disaster, it can be useful to engage in activities that help people regain a sense of control. This will help support the healing and recovery process.
- **Asking for help and seeking resources.** Resourceful people will get needed help more quickly if they know how to ask questions, are creative in their thinking about situations, are good problem solvers and communicators, and have a good social network to reach out to.
- **Seeing yourself as resilient.** After a disaster many people may feel helpless and powerless, especially when there has been vast damage to the community. Being able to see yourself as resilient, rather than as helpless or as a victim, can help build psychological resilience.
- **Coping with stress in healthy ways.** People get feelings of pleasure and self-worth from doing things well. Strategies that use positive and meaningful ways to cope are better than those which can be harmful such as drinking too much or smoking.
- **Helping others and finding positive meaning in life.** Positive emotions like gratitude, joy, kindness, love, and contentment can come from helping others. Acts of generosity can add meaning and purpose to your life, even in the face of tragedy.

Resilient individuals are able to:
- Care for themselves and others day-to-day and during emergency situations
- Actively support their neighborhoods, workplaces, and communities to recover after disaster
- Be confident and hopeful about overcoming present and future difficulties
- Get needed resources more effectively and quickly
- Be physically and mentally healthier and have overall lower recovery expenses and service needs
- Miss fewer days of work
- Maintain stable family and social connections
- Re-establish routines more quickly, which helps children and adults alike

WAYS TO STRENGTHEN RESILIENCE

You can build your resilience by taking care of your health, managing stress, and being an active participant in the life of your community. For example, try to:
- Develop coping skills and practice stress management activities, such as yoga, exercise, and meditation.
- Eat healthily and exercise.
- Get plenty of sleep.
- Maintain social connections to people and groups that are meaningful for you.
- Volunteer in your community.
- Get training in first aid, cardiopulmonary resuscitation (CPR), computer emergency response team (CERT), and psychological first aid (PFA).
- Create evacuation and family reunification plans.
- Make a disaster kit and stock supplies to shelter in place for up to three days.
- Find things that bring you pleasure and enjoyment such as reading a book or watching a movie, writing in a journal, or engaging in an art activity.

DOES INDIVIDUAL RESILIENCE HELP BUILD COMMUNITY RESILIENCE?

Yes! Individual resilience is important to community resilience in that healthy people make for a healthier community. Healthy communities are better able to manage and recover from disasters and other emergencies.

Section 45.2 | Fostering Resilience in Children and Adolescents

This section contains text excerpted from the following sources: Text in this section begins with excerpts from "Childhood Resilience," Substance Abuse and Mental Health Services Administration (SAMHSA), July 31, 2019; Text under the heading "Positive Adolescent Mental Health: Resilience" is excerpted from "Positive Adolescent Mental Health: Resilience," U.S. Department of Health and Human Services (HHS), October 28, 2016. Reviewed August 2020.

We cannot "make" children resilient, but we can shine a light on those qualities and skills that help them develop key elements of resiliency. Ann Masten, one of the foremost researchers of resilience in children, writes, "Resilience does not come from rare and special qualities, but from the everyday magic of ordinary, normative human resources in the minds, brains, and bodies of children, in their families and relationships, and in their communities." This "ordinary magic" means that children will be more able to adapt to adversity and threats when their basic human systems are nurtured and supported.

FACTORS THAT CONTRIBUTE TO CHILDHOOD RESILIENCE
Cognitive Development/Problem-Solving Skills

As a species, we have been solving problems since the beginning of time. Watch a child play and you will see that her/his problem-solving skills are nearly always at work. Infants attempt to soothe themselves by figuring out how to put their thumbs in their mouths or crying for a caregiver. Toddlers try to fit shapes into shape sorters. As children mature, the problems they solve get more complex. Solving problems engage our prefrontal cortex, sometimes called the "thinking brain," which is the seat of our executive function. During times of stress and trauma, this part of our brain is typically shut down so that our body can respond to the threats it is facing. By helping children engage in problem-solving activities, they not only gain a sense of self-efficacy and mastery, they also re-engage the parts of their brain that may have been offline. Because the neural pathways of young brains are still being wired, the more we can engage and reinforce healthy pathways, the better. Developing problem-solving skills also helps children with self-regulation skills, another key quality that fosters resilience.

Self-Regulation

Self-regulation is the ability to control oneself in a variety of ways. Infants develop regular sleep-wake patterns. Schoolchildren learn to raise their hands and wait patiently to be called on rather than shouting out an answer. College students concentrate for hours on a research paper, delaying the gratification that might come with being outdoors on a sunny day. Self-regulation has been identified as "the cornerstone" of child development. In the seminal publication *From Neurons to Neighborhoods*, experts conclude, "Development may be viewed as an increased capacity for self-regulation, seen particularly in the child's ability to function more independently in a personal and social context." It involves working memory, the ability to focus on a goal, tolerance for frustration, and controlling and expressing one's emotions appropriately and in context. Self-regulation is the key for academic and social success and plays a significant role in mental-health outcomes—all things that can be a challenge for children experiencing homelessness and other stressors.

Relationships with Caring Adults

Ideally, we form close attachment relationships with our primary caregiver(s) beginning at birth. As we get older, those relationships extend to teachers, neighbors, family, friends, coaches, and others. Disrupted attachment relationships can be devastating for young children because they are still developing an internal working model of what relationships look like and because they rely so intensively on their caregivers to get their basic needs met.

By developing relationships with caring adults, whether they be parents, family members, coaches, teachers, or neighbors, children learn about healthy relationships—ones that are consistent, predictable, and safe. They receive guidance, comfort, and mentoring.

PLAY: A KEY STRATEGY FOR DEVELOPING RESILIENCE

What strategies can we use to draw out children's resilience? The short answer is playing. According to the Life Is Good Playmakers Blog, "Children who grow up afraid do not learn how to play. They learn how to survive." One of our jobs then becomes to draw out children's natural playfulness, which gives them an opportunity to discover, learn, and heal. As the iconic Fred Rogers tells us, "Play gives children a chance to practice what they are learning. They have to play with what they know to be true in order to find out more, and then they can use what they learn in new forms of play." We can create play experiences for children of all ages that give them ways to engage in solving problems, develop self-regulation skills, and form relationships. Here are some ideas:

- "Simon Says" helps children practice several self-regulation skills (e.g., working memory and inhibitory control).
- Legos, blocks, and other tactile toys give children opportunities to solve problems and focus on a goal ("I want to build a tower. How can I build the tower really high without it falling?"). If they are playing with an adult (especially one who lets the child direct the play), they are also building a relationship.
- Breathing exercises and body work (yoga, stretching)
- Reading books, playing games, and having conversations about identifying emotions
- Letting children talk aloud (and/or hear you talk aloud) about solving a problem. What are the pros and cons of possible solutions?
- Dancing, singing, listening to music, and playing musical instruments and experimenting with speed

(fast song, slow song), volume (sing loudly, sing quietly), and breath (play your instrument and hold the note as long as you can...now try making short, staccato notes)

- Any activity that strengthens the relationship between the child and her/his primary caregiver

POSITIVE ADOLESCENT MENTAL HEALTH: RESILIENCE

"Resilient" adolescents are those who have managed to cope effectively, even in the face of stress and other difficult circumstances, and are poised to enter adulthood with a good chance of positive mental health. A number of factors promote resilience in adolescents—among the most important are caring relationships with adults and an easy-going disposition. Adolescents themselves can use a number of strategies, including exercising regularly, to reduce stress and promote resilience. Schools and communities are also recognizing the importance of resilience and general "emotional intelligence" in adolescents' lives—a growing number of courses and community programs focus on adolescents' social-emotional learning and coping skills.

Chapter 46 | Social Connectedness and Mental Health

Strong, healthy relationships are important throughout your life. Your social ties with family members, friends, neighbors, coworkers, and others impact your mental, emotional, and even physical well-being.

"We cannot underestimate the power of a relationship in helping to promote well-being," says the National Institutes of Health (NIH) psychologist and relationship expert Dr. Valerie Maholmes. Studies have found that having a variety of social relationships may help reduce stress and heart-related risks. Strong social ties are even linked to a longer life. On the other hand, loneliness and social isolation are linked to poorer health, depression, and increased risk of early death.

As a child you learn the social skills you need to form and maintain relationships with others. But at any age, you can learn ways to improve your relationships.

The NIH funds research to find out what causes unhealthy relationship behavior. Researchers have created community, family, and school-based programs to help people learn to have healthier relationships. These programs also help prevent abuse and violence toward others.

This chapter includes text excerpted from "Building Social Bonds: Connections That Promote Well-Being," *NIH News in Health*, National Institutes of Health (NIH), April 2018.

WHAT IS HEALTHY RELATIONSHIP?

Every relationship exists on a spectrum from healthy to unhealthy to abusive. One sign of a healthy relationship is feeling good about yourself around your partner, family member, or friend. You feel safe talking about how you feel. You listen to each other. You feel valued, and you trust each other.

"It is important for people to recognize and be aware of any time where there is a situation in their relationship that does not feel right to them or that makes them feel less than who they are," Maholmes advises.

It is normal for people to disagree with each other. But, conflicts should not turn into personal attacks. In a healthy relationship, you can disagree without hurting each other and make decisions together.

"No relationship should be based on that power dynamic where someone is constantly putting the other partner down," Maholmes says.

If you grew up in a family with abuse, it may be hard as an adult to know what healthy relationship is. Abuse may feel normal to you. There are several kinds of abuse, including physical, sexual, and verbal or emotional. Hurting with words, neglect, and withholding affection are examples of verbal or emotional abuse.

In an unhealthy or abusive relationship, your partner may blame you for feeling bad about something they did or said. They may tell you that you are too sensitive. Putting you down diminishes you and keeps them in control.

In a healthy relationship, however, if you tell your partner that something they said hurt your feelings, they feel bad for hurting you. They try not to do it again.

Abuse in an intimate relationship is called "domestic" or "intimate partner violence." This type of violence involves a pattern of behaviors used by one person to maintain power and control over someone who they are married to, living with, or dating now or in the past. A pattern means it happens over and over.

In an unhealthy or abusive relationship, you may not be allowed to spend time with family, friends, and others in your social network. "One of the signs that is really important in relationships where there is intimate partner violence is that the partner that is being abused is slowly being isolated from family and friends and social networks," Maholmes says. "Those social networks are protective factors."

SOCIAL TIES PROTECT

Studies have shown that certain factors seem to protect people from forming unhealthy relationships over their lifetime. The protection starts early in life. The NIH-supported research has shown that the quality of an infant's emotional bond with a parent can have long-lasting positive or negative effects on the ability to develop healthy relationships.

"The early bond has implications that go well beyond the first years of life," says Dr. Grazyna Kochanska, an NIH-funded family relationships researcher at the University of Iowa. The goal of Kochanska's research projects is to understand the long-term effects of that early bond and to help children develop along positive pathways and avoid paths toward antisocial behaviors.

A family that functions well is central to a child's development. Parents can help children learn how to listen, set appropriate boundaries, and resolve conflicts. Parents teach children by example how to consider other people's feelings and act in ways to benefit others.

Secure emotional bonds help children and teens develop trust and self-esteem. They can then venture out of the family to form other social connections, like healthy friendships. In turn, healthy friendships reduce the risk of a child becoming emotionally distressed or engaging in antisocial behaviors.

On the other hand, having an unhealthy relationship in the family, including neglect and abuse, puts a child at risk for future unhealthy relationships.

"One caring adult can make a huge difference in the life of kids whose family structures may not be ideal or whose early life is characterized by abuse and neglect," says Dr. Jennie Noll of the Center for Healthy Children at Pennsylvania State University. "That caring adult could be an older sibling, or a parent, or someone else in the family, a teacher—the kind of people who have a large influence in communicating to the child that they matter and that they are safe, and that they have a place to go when they are needing extra support."

Healthy friendships and activities outside of the home or classroom can play protective roles during childhood, too. In fact, everyone in a community can help support the development of healthy connections. Adults can serve as good role models for children, whether the children are their own or those they choose to mentor.

HELPING AND GETTING HELP

At any age, your relationships matter. Having healthy relationships with others starts with liking yourself. Learn what makes you happy. Treat yourself well. Know that you deserve to be treated well by others.

Having an unhealthy or abusive relationship can really hurt. The connection may be good some of the time. You may love and need the person who hurts you. After being abused, you may feel you do not deserve to be in a healthy, loving relationship.

With help, you can work on your relationship. Or, sometimes in an abusive relationship, you may be advised to get out. Either way, others can help.

If you or a friend needs help with an unhealthy relationship, contact the National Domestic Violence Hotline at www.thehotline.org or 800-799-SAFE. If you know a child who may need help, find resources at the Child Welfare Information Gateway at www.childwelfare.gov.

Chapter 47 | Behavioral and Mental-Health Needs in Older Adults

Mental-health issues are exceedingly common and affect approximately one in four people. Contrary to popular belief, mental-health issues are not a normal part of aging, rather it should be treated as a serious condition. As a person becomes old, life changes, including illness and retirement, making them more vulnerable to mental-health problems. The worldwide population is aging rapidly, and the need for behavioral and mental-health services are constantly increasing. Studies show that between 2015 and 2050, the proportion of the elderly people in the global population, which is 12 percent, will rise close to 22 percent.

SIGNIFICANT BEHAVIORAL AND MENTAL-HEALTH PROBLEMS IN ELDERLY ADULTS

Due to limited access to mental healthcare resources, behavioral and mental-health problems are becoming more common among older adults. Psychologists are trying to address these mental-health needs for older patients by studying and treating behavioral issues related to:

- Aging
- Bereavement
- Loss of independence and mobility

"Behavioral and Mental-Health Needs in Older Adults," © 2020 Omnigraphics. Reviewed August 2020.

- Living in a long-term health facility
- Declining physical health

These problems often result in deteriorating mental health and neurological disorders among older adults.

The following are some of the most common behavioral and mental-health issues that older adults suffer from:

Substance Abuse

Substance-use disorders (SUDs) are some of the most commonly overlooked behavioral health issues faced by older adults. More than 1.5 million American adults over 65 years of age are reported to have SUDs, according to a 2017 survey by Substance Abuse and Mental Health Services Administration (SAMHSA). Also, 5.7 million adults 65 years of age and older had alcohol-use disorder (AUD). It is also important to consider that SUD exists with comorbid psychiatric disorders in older adults such as depression, sleep disorder, cognitive impairment, and such disorders lead to greater suicide risk.

Depression and Suicidal Ideation

Depression among older adults is known to be lesser than it is among youngsters; however, the consequences prove to be just as significant. Older adults may experience depression associated with reduced quality of life, cognitive decline, disability, and certain medical conditions. Around 37 percent of nursing home residents are known to suffer from depression. Suicide ideation is a vital consequence of depression for older people, and they do not exhibit any expressive warning signs when compared to younger adults with suicidal thoughts. Older adults account for 13 percent of the U.S. population, but they make up 20 percent of people who commit suicide.

Anxiety Disorders

One of the most common behavioral health problems in older adults is generalized anxiety disorder (GAD), and around 50 percent of them develop symptoms only in later life. Other types of anxiety disorders, except for the fear of falling, usually develop at a young age. Similar to depression, anxiety is one of the most prevalent mental issues, and most older adults diagnosed with depression also suffer from anxiety. Anxiety is often left unnoticed in older adults since they focus more on physical symptoms of illness that generally occur during old age. A lifetime diagnosis of anxiety has not been reported by more than 90 percent of adults aged 50 or older.

Agitation

Incidents of agitation or aggression among older adults are usually caused by major neurocognitive disorders and delirium, which can potentially become a life-threatening emergency. This is usually triggered by pain, adverse medication reactions, withdrawal symptoms, psychosis, and mania. Agitation symptoms include various verbal and physical behaviors such as yelling, pacing, hitting, and kicking. De-escalation techniques, such as reassurance by a family member or a familiar caregiver can help calm them down during such times. If this approach does not work, emergency medication can be used to make them relax so that further treatment can be administered to alleviate the agitation symptoms.

Psychosis

Psychosis is a mental condition that causes a person to lose touch with reality, resulting in delusions, disoriented speech and behavior, or hallucinations. Delirium and dementia are the two most common causes of psychosis in older patients, followed by mood-related psychoses, especially psychotic depression and psychotic mania. Psychotic depression is characterized by signs of depression and delusions of guilt or persecution and sometimes accompanied by hallucinations. Psychotic mania has similar symptoms, except delusions of grandiose and religious nature, along with a few other signs such as pressured speech, reduced sleep, and less concentration or disorganization.

Dementia

The irreversible deterioration of a person's intellectual ability, along with emotional disturbances, is referred to as dementia. This affects about 30 percent of Americans above 85 years of age and 7 percent of those above 65. Dementia is often accompanied by depression, anxiety, and paranoia. The most common cause of dementia is Alzheimer disease, which affects 2.6 to 4.5 million Americans aged above 65 years old. Alzheimer disease cases are found to be doubling every five years among people 65 to 85 years of age and older.

TREATMENT AND CARE STRATEGIES

The behavioral and mental health of older adults can be enhanced by creating an environment that can help them stay physically and mentally healthy. The mental health of older adults can be improved based on the following strategies:

- Providing them with the necessary security and freedom
- Offering social support for both older adults and their caregivers, if any
- Creating awareness and programs designed to prevent and deal with elder abuse
- Health and social programs for the rural older population and older patients with chronic mental or physical illness

Healthcare providers must also be prepared to meet the specific requirements of older people, such as:

- Providing training for healthcare professionals to care for older adults
- Formulating sustainable policies for long-term and palliative/hospice care
- Establishing age-friendly assistance services and environments
- Preventing and treating age-related chronic illnesses such as neurological, mental, and SUD

BEHAVIORAL AND MENTAL-HEALTH NEED INTERVENTIONS

It is essential to promptly recognize and treat mental-health concerns in older adults using both psychosocial interventions and

348

medications. There is no medication to cure certain mental ill-nesses, such as dementia completely. However, there are ways to support and improve the lives of the person affected, their families, and caregivers:

- Early diagnosis of the condition to promote optimal management and treatment
- Recognizing and treating comorbid physical illnesses
- Identifying and managing challenging behaviors
- Providing long-term support and training to caregivers
- Improving mental healthcare in the community

A supportive legislative environment that is based on a set of internationally accepted human rights standards is necessary to ensure the proper level of care for people with mental illness and their caregivers.

HOW TO FOSTER BETTER BEHAVIORAL AND MENTAL HEALTH

There are many effective treatments and self-help techniques that can help improve an older adult's mental health. Given below are a few steps that can be followed to promote behavioral and mental health among older adults.

- **Staying connected.** Isolation can often lead to mental issues; therefore, it is necessary to keep in touch with loved ones and increase social connections. This can be done by enrolling in a new class or starting a hobby.
- **Being productive.** Staying active, especially with outdoor activities, boosts the general mood and enhances physical as well as mental health. It is essential to have a regular activity to keep one occupied, such as gardening, walking, cycling, or yoga.
- **Eat healthy.** Having a healthy diet can have a positive effect on both physical and mental health. Eat a balanced diet and stay hydrated while avoiding high-sugar food and drinks and excessive alcohol.
- **Get sufficient sleep.** Daily routines can be modified to better match with the sleep schedule and learning

relaxation techniques such as breathing exercises can help one feel calm and get adequate sleep.

- **Have a sense of purpose.** It is necessary to have a sense of purpose in life, especially for older people, so they can prevent negative thoughts about life. For instance, volunteering can make people feel like they are helping a cause, thereby improving their mental health.

Mental health and well-being of older adults should be considered a vital aspect of American healthcare. Oftentimes, symptoms of depression and anxiety in older Americans are left untreated since they occur simultaneously with life events (losing a loved one) or medical conditions that are common in old age.

References

1. "Behavioral Health Needs of Older Adults in the Emergency Department," National Center for Biotechnology Information, June 15, 2018.
2. "Older Adults and Mental Health," Independent Age, April 3, 2020.
3. "Growing Mental and Behavioral Health Concerns Facing Older Americans," American Psychological Association (APA), August 24, 2018.
4. "Mental Health of Older Adults," World Health Organization (WHO), December 12, 2017.

Chapter 48 | Financial Assistance for Treating Mental-Health Problems

Approximately 1 in 5 U.S. adolescents experience mental disorders with severe impairment, and 1 in 5 U.S. adults (excluding adolescents) had mild-to-severe symptoms of mental illness in the past year. However, every year, many adolescents and adults with mental illness go untreated. Recent data suggests that half of the adults who felt the need for mental-health treatment but did not receive it within that year reported not being able to afford treatment as a major reason for not receiving care. However, this data collection occurred before the implementation of the Affordable Care Act (ACA), so the number of adults who feel the need for treatment but do not receive it may be reduced in the future.

Mental-health facilities that offer services at no charge or use a sliding-fee scale serve as a safety net for those individuals who need but cannot afford to pay for these services. Although the literature in this area is sparse, a few studies have examined the availability of free general health clinics and the organizational structure of these clinics. In general, free clinics were defined in the available studies as nonprofit entities that offer uninsured and underserved individuals access to reduced cost or free healthcare services. One available survey of free general health clinics found that about one-third of these clinics also offered mental-health treatment. However,

This chapter includes text excerpted from "Availability of Payment Assistance for Mental Health Services in U.S. Mental Health Treatment Facilities," Substance Abuse and Mental Health Services Administration (SAMHSA), March 23, 2016. Reviewed August 2020.

mental-health services may be provided not just in free general health clinics, but also by specialty mental-health facilities. Studies that focus on the national availability of mental-health facilities that provide mental-health services either for free or with payment assistance are limited. Estimates of the number of mental-health facilities nationwide that provide mental-health services without charge or with some financial aid are not available. This knowledge is important because the affordability of mental-health services may be a factor in individuals' willingness to seek treatment, and the availability of a wide range of different healthcare settings for mental-health service delivery may improve access to treatment. This report examines the availability of mental-health treatment services provided at no charge or using a sliding-fee scale in the U.S. mental-health treatment facilities.

The National Mental Health Services Survey (N-MHSS) is an annual survey of all known mental-health treatment facilities in the United States, both public and private. The N-MHSS is conducted by the Substance Abuse and Mental Health Services Administration (SAMHSA) and is designed to collect data on the location, characteristics, and use of mental-health treatment facilities throughout the 50 states, the District of Columbia, and other U.S. jurisdictions.

The 2010 N-MHSS is the most recent available analytic data file and is used in this study. The final 2010 N-MHSS facility universe included 16,197 mental-health treatment facilities, of which 12,186 were eligible for the survey. Of the 11,118 (91.2%) eligible facilities that responded to the 2010 N-MHSS, 10,374 were included in the N-MHSS main findings report and data files. The 10,374 facilities included 1,235 facilities that completed an abbreviated follow-up questionnaire (basic facility information and client counts) and 9,139 facilities that completed all sections of the questionnaire, including basic facility information, services characteristics, and client counts. This report focuses on the 8,938 facilities that completed all sections of the survey questionnaire and responded to the two items on payment assistance. Because the N-MHSS involves censuses and actual counts rather than estimates, statistical significance and confidence intervals are not applicable. The differences between proportions mentioned in the text of this report have

Financial Assistance for Treating Mental-Health Problems

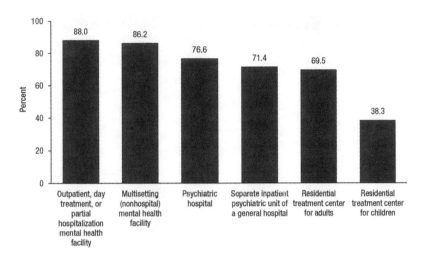

Figure 48.1. Mental-Health Treatment Facilities Offering Payment Assistance, by Facility Type: 2010 N-MHSS (Source: SAMHSA, National Mental Health Services Survey (N-MHSS), 2010)

Note: Based on 8,938 facilities that completed all sections of the survey questionnaire and responded to the two items on payment assistance.
Note: Percentages may not sum to 100.0 percent due to rounding.

Cohen's h effect size > 0.20, indicating that they are considered to be meaningful.

DESCRIPTION OF MENTAL-HEALTH TREATMENT FACILITIES THAT OFFER PAYMENT ASSISTANCE

The availability of payment assistance (i.e., services available at no charge or with a sliding-fee scale) differed by type of treatment facility. Payment assistance was offered in 88.0 percent of outpatient mental-health centers, 86.2 percent of multi-setting mental-health facilities, 76.6 percent of psychiatric hospitals, and 71.4 percent of general hospitals with separate psychiatric units (Figure 48.1.). Multi-setting mental-health facilities are "facilities that provide outpatient and residential mental-health services and are not classified as a psychiatric or general hospital with a separate psychiatric unit or as residential treatment centers (RTCs)." Among residential treatment centers (RTCs) for adults, 69.5 percent offered payment

Characteristic	Number	Percent
Facility operation		
Private for-profit organization	412	49.6
Private nonprofit organization	4,783	79.6
State mental health agency (SMHA)	612	94.9
Local, county, or municipal government	785	94.7
Other	557	89.0
Primary treatment focus		
Mental health services	5,259	78.6
Mix of mental health and substance abuse services	1,890	84.1
Other languages		
Spanish or other languages spoken by staff providing services	2,964	85.4
Age group of patients/clients accepted by facility		
Youth (aged 17 or younger)	4,602	81.0
Adults (18 to 64)	6,385	83.4
Seniors (65 or older)	5,683	84.5
Urbanicity		
Large metropolitan counties	1,682	78.3
Large fringe metro	1,327	77.4
Medium metro counties	1,287	78.6
Small metro counties	813	78.7
Micropolitan	1,103	81.6
Noncore	934	89.0
Region		
Northeast	1,562	77.4
Midwest	1,900	79.6
South	2,170	81.2
West	1,517	81.6

Figure 48.2. Characteristics of Mental-Health Treatment Facilities Offering Payment Assistance: 2010 N-MHSS (Source: SAMHSA, National Mental Health Services Survey (N-MHSS), 2010)

Note: Based on 8,938 facilities that offered payment assistance. Facilities with unknown description were excluded from the analysis.
Note: Urbanicity based on the 2006 National Center for Health Statistics Urban-Rural Classification Scheme for Counties (www.cdc.gov/nchs/data_access/urban_rural.htm).

assistance. In contrast, slightly more than one-third of RTCs for children offered payment assistance (38.3%).

More than three-fourths of facilities operated by private non-profit organizations (79.6%) and almost all facilities operated by state mental-health agencies (94.9%) or local, county, or municipal governments (94.7%) offered payment assistance. In contrast, about half of the facilities operated by private for-profit organizations offered payment assistance (49.6%). Of the facilities that offered services in Spanish or other languages, 85.4 percent provided payment assistance. Payment assistance was available across a majority of U.S. regions but was available in more facilities located in the most rural, or "noncore," counties (89.0%) than facilities located in more urban counties (range of 77.4 to 81.6%).

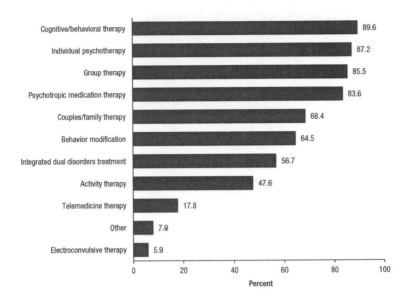

Figure 48.3. Mental-Health Treatment Approaches Provided in Facilities Offering Payment Assistance: 2010 NMHSS (Source: SAMHSA, National Mental Health Services Survey (N-MHSS), 2010)

Note: Based on 8,938 facilities that offered payment assistance. Facilities with unknown treatment approaches were excluded from the analysis.

TREATMENT APPROACHES PROVIDED IN MENTAL-HEALTH TREATMENT FACILITIES THAT OFFERED PAYMENT ASSISTANCE

A majority of the facilities that offered payment assistance (either service at no charge or with a sliding-fee scale) provided cognitive/behavioral therapy (89.6%), individual psychotherapy (87.2%), group therapy (85.5%), and psychotropic medication therapy (83.6%; Figure 48.3.). More than half of facilities that offered payment assistance provided couples/family therapy (68.4%), behavior modification (64.5%), and integrated dual disorders treatment (56.7%).

Chapter 49 | **Anxiety Disorder and Disability Accommodations**

Chapter Contents

Section 49.1 | Anxiety Disorder and the Americans with Disabilities Act

This section includes text excerpted from "Depression, PTSD, and Other Mental Health Conditions in the Workplace: Your Legal Rights," U.S. Equal Employment Opportunity Commission (EEOC), December 12, 2016. Reviewed August 2020.

If you have depression, posttraumatic stress disorder (PTSD), or another mental-health condition, you are protected against discrimination and harassment at work because of your condition, you have workplace privacy rights, and you may have a legal right to get reasonable accommodations that can help you perform and keep your job. The following questions and answers briefly explain these rights, which are provided by the Americans with Disabilities Act (ADA). You may also have additional rights under other laws not discussed here, such as the Family and Medical Leave Act (FMLA) and various medical insurance laws.

IS YOUR EMPLOYER ALLOWED TO FIRE YOUR BECAUSE YOU HAVE A MENTAL-HEALTH CONDITION?

No. It is illegal for an employer to discriminate against you simply because you have a mental-health condition. This includes firing you, rejecting you for a job or promotion, or forcing you to take leave.

An employer does not have to hire or keep people in jobs the cannot perform, or employ people who pose a "direct threat" to safety (a significant risk of substantial harm to self or others). But, an employer cannot rely on myths or stereotypes about your mental-health condition when deciding whether you can perform a job or whether you pose a safety risk. Before an employer can reject you for a job based on your condition, it must have objective evidence that you cannot perform your job duties, or that you would create a significant safety risk, even with a reasonable accommodation.

ARE YOU ALLOWED TO KEEP YOUR CONDITION PRIVATE?

In most situations, you can keep your condition private. An employer is only allowed to ask medical questions (including questions about mental health) in four situations:

359

- When you ask for a reasonable accommodation.
- After it has made you a job offer, but before employment begins, as long as everyone entering the same job category is asked the same questions.
- When it is engaging in affirmative action for people with disabilities (such as an employer tracking the disability status of its applicant pool in order to assess its recruitment and hiring efforts, or a public sector employer considering whether special hiring rules may apply), in which case you may choose whether to respond.
- On the job, when there is objective evidence that you may be unable to do your job or that you may pose a safety risk because of your condition.

You also may need to discuss your condition to establish eligibility for benefits under other laws, such as the Family and Medical Leave Act (FMLA). If you do talk about your condition, the employer cannot discriminate against you, and it must keep the information confidential, even from coworkers. (If you wish to discuss your condition with coworkers, you may choose to do so.)

WHAT IF YOUR MENTAL-HEALTH CONDITION COULD AFFECT YOUR JOB PERFORMANCE?

You may have a legal right to a reasonable accommodation that would help you do your job. A reasonable accommodation is some type of change in the way things are normally done at work. Just a few examples of possible accommodations include altered break and work schedules (e.g., scheduling work around therapy appointments), quiet office space or devices that create a quiet work environment, changes in supervisory methods (e.g., written instructions from a supervisor who usually does not provide them), specific shift assignments, and permission to work from home.

You can get a reasonable accommodation for any mental-health condition that would, if left untreated, "substantially limit" your ability to concentrate, interact with others, communicate, eat, sleep, care for yourself, regulate your thoughts or emotions, or do any other "major life activity." (You do not need to actually stop treatment to get the accommodation.)

Your condition does not need to be permanent or severe to be "substantially limiting." It may qualify by, for example, making activities more difficult, uncomfortable, or time-consuming to perform compared to the way that most people perform them. If your symptoms come and go, what matters is how limiting they would be when the symptoms are present. Mental-health conditions like major depression, PTSD, bipolar disorder, schizophrenia, and obsessive-compulsive disorder (OCD) should easily qualify, and many others will qualify as well.

HOW CAN YOU GET A REASONABLE ACCOMMODATION?

Ask for one. Tell a supervisor, HR manager, or other appropriate person that you need a change at work because of a medical condition. You may ask for an accommodation at any time. Because an employer does not have to excuse poor job performance, even if it was caused by a medical condition or the side effects of medication, it is generally better to get a reasonable accommodation before any problems occur or become worse. (Many people choose to wait to ask for accommodation until after they receive a job offer, however, because it is very hard to prove illegal discrimination that takes place before a job offer.) You do not need to have a particular accommodation in mind, but you can ask for something specific.

WHAT WILL HAPPEN AFTER YOU ASK FOR A REASONABLE ACCOMMODATION?

Your employer may ask you to put your request in writing, and to generally describe your condition and how it affects your work. The employer also may ask you to submit a letter from your healthcare provider documenting that you have a mental-health condition, and that you need an accommodation because of it. If you do not want the employer to know your specific diagnosis, it may be enough to provide documentation that describes your condition more generally (e.g., by stating, that you have an "anxiety disorder"). Your employer also might ask your healthcare provider whether particular accommodations would meet your needs. You can help your healthcare provider understand the law of reasonable accommodation by bringing a copy of the Equal Employment Opportunity Commission's (EEOC) publication *The Mental-Health Provider's Role in a Client's Request for a Reasonable Accommodation at Work* to your appointment.

If a reasonable accommodation would help you to do your job, your employer must give you one unless the accommodation involves significant difficulty or expense. If more than one accommodation would work, the employer can choose which one to give you. Your employer cannot legally fire you, or refuse to hire or promote you, because you asked for a reasonable accommodation or because you need one. They also cannot charge you for the cost of the accommodation.

WHAT IF THERE IS NO WAY YOU CAN DO YOUR REGULAR JOB, EVEN WITH AN ACCOMMODATION?

If you cannot perform all the essential functions of your job to normal standards and have no paid leave available, you still may be entitled to unpaid leave as a reasonable accommodation if that leave will help you get to a point where you can perform those functions. You may also qualify for leave under the FMLA, which is enforced by the United States Department of Labor. More information about this law can be found at www.dol.gov/whd/fmla.

If you are permanently unable to do your regular job, you may ask your employer to reassign you to a job that you can do as a reasonable accommodation, if one is available.

WHAT IF YOU ARE BEING HARASSED BECAUSE OF YOUR CONDITION?

Harassment based on a disability is not allowed under the ADA. You should tell your employer about any harassment if you want the employer to stop the problem. Follow your employer's reporting procedures if there are any. If you report the harassment, your employer is legally required to take action to prevent it from occurring in the future.

WHAT SHOULD YOU DO IF YOU THINK THAT YOUR RIGHTS HAVE BEEN VIOLATED?

The EEOC can help you decide what to do next, and conduct an investigation if you decide to file a charge of discrimination. Because you must file a charge within 180 days of the alleged violation in order to take further legal action (or 300 days if the employer is also covered by a state or local employment discrimination law), it is best to begin the process early. It is illegal for your employer to retaliate against you for contacting the EEOC or filing a charge.

Section 49.2 | Accommodating Employees with Anxiety Disorder

This section includes text excerpted from "Maximizing Productivity: Accommodations for Employees with Psychiatric Disabilities," U.S. Department of Labor (DOL), April 6, 2006. Reviewed August 2020.

A psychiatric disability can impact various aspects of an individual's life, including the ability to achieve maximum productivity in the workplace. The National Institute of Mental Health (NIMH) estimates that one in five people will experience a psychiatric disability in their lifetime, and one in four Americans currently knows someone who has a psychiatric disability. It is likely that most employers have at least one employee with a psychiatric disability.

Under the Americans with Disabilities Act (ADA) and other nondiscrimination laws, most employers must provide "reasonable accommodations" to qualified employees with disabilities. Many employers are aware of different types of accommodations for people with physical and communication disabilities, but they may be less familiar with accommodations for employees with disabilities that are not visible, such as psychiatric disabilities. Over the last few years, increasing numbers of employers have expressed a desire and need for information and ideas on accommodations for employees with psychiatric disabilities.

Reasonable accommodations are adjustments to a work setting that make it possible for qualified employees with disabilities to perform the essential functions of their jobs. The majority of accommodations can be made for minimal (if any) cost and a small investment of time and planning. Moreover, effective accommodations can be good for business. They help employees return to work more quickly after disability or medical leave, eliminate costs due to lost productivity and can be key to recruiting and retaining qualified employees.

Not all employees with psychiatric disabilities need accommodations to perform their jobs. For those who do, it is important to remember that the process of developing and implementing accommodations is individualized and should begin with input from the employee. Accommodations vary, just as people's strengths, work environments and job duties vary.

Below are examples of accommodations that have helped employees with psychiatric disabilities to more effectively perform their jobs. The list below does not include all possible accommodations, but it is a good starting point and provides some of the most effective and frequently used workplace accommodations. For example:

- **Flexible workplace.** Telecommuting and/or working from home.
- **Scheduling.** Part-time work hours, job sharing, adjustments in the start or end of work hours, compensation time and/or "make up" of missed time.
- **Leave.** Sick leave for reasons related to mental health, flexible use of vacation time, additional unpaid or administrative leave for treatment or recovery, leaves of absence and/or use of occasional leave (a few hours at a time) for therapy and other related appointments.
- **Breaks.** Breaks according to individual needs rather than a fixed schedule, more frequent breaks and/or greater flexibility in scheduling breaks, provision of backup coverage during breaks, and telephone breaks during work hours to call professionals and others needed for support.
- **Other policies.** Beverages and/or food permitted at workstations, if necessary, to mitigate the side effects of medications, on-site job coaches.

MODIFICATIONS

- Reduction and/or removal of distractions in the work area
- Addition of room dividers, partitions or other soundproofing or visual barriers between workspaces to reduce noise or visual distractions
- Private offices or private space enclosures
- Office/work space location away from noisy machinery
- Reduction of workplace noise that can be adjusted (such as telephone volume)
- Increased natural lighting or full spectrum lighting
- Music (with headset) to block out distractions

EQUIPMENT/TECHNOLOGY

- Tape recorders for recording/reviewing meetings and training sessions
- "White noise" or environmental sound machines
- Handheld electronic organizers, software calendars and organizer programs
- Remote job coaching, laptop computers, personal digital assistants and office computer access via remote locations
- Software that minimizes computerized distractions, such as pop-up screens

JOB DUTIES

- Modification or removal of nonessential job duties or restructuring of the job to include only the essential job functions
- Division of large assignments into smaller tasks and goals
- Additional assistance and/or time for orientation activities, training and learning job tasks, and new responsibilities
- Additional training or modified training materials

MANAGEMENT/SUPERVISION

- Implementation of flexible and supportive supervision style; positive reinforcement and feedback; adjustments

in level of supervision or structure such as more
frequent meetings to help prioritize tasks; and open
communication with supervisors regarding performance
and work expectations

- Additional forms of communication and/or written and
visual tools, including communication of assignments
and instructions in the employee's preferred learning style
(written, verbal, e-mail, demonstration); creation and
implementation of written tools such as daily "to-do" lists,
step-by-step checklists, written (in addition to verbal)
instructions and typed minutes of meetings
- Regularly scheduled meetings (weekly or monthly) with
employees to discuss workplace issues and productivity,
including annual discussions as part of performance
appraisals to assess abilities and discuss promotional
opportunities
- Development of strategies to deal with problems before
they arise
- Written work agreements that include any agreed upon
accommodations, long-term and short-term goals,
expectations of responsibilities and consequences of not
meeting performance standards
- Education of all employees about their right to
accommodations
- Relevant training for all employees, including coworkers
and supervisory staff

Section 49.3 | **A Support Person as an Accommodation**

WHO IS A SUPPORT PERSON?

A support person is someone of an employee's choice who can attend a meeting along with them to provide emotional support and reassurance. They are not to be confused with advocates. Anyone can be a support person, be it a colleague, family member, friend, or a lawyer.

WHEN IS A SUPPORT PERSON NEEDED?

A support person as an accommodation is needed and helpful for people with various disabilities and impairments, namely those with mental-health impairments, learning and intellectual disabilities, brain injuries, attention deficit hyperactivity disorder (ADHD), and autism. These individuals can primarily benefit from having a support person on the job.

Similarly, people who have difficulty managing emotions and stress or often affected by anxiety find having a support person exceedingly comforting, encouraging, and help improve a person's reaction in situations that may aggravate their mental-health issue.

A SUPPORT PERSON FOR THE WORKPLACE

A workplace always has issues of conflicts or disagreements, and a disability can add to the stress and worry of a person. For example, if a person with an anxiety disorder is about to have a meeting with an employer, the situation can instigate more worry. In such situations, bringing a support person can help ease this tension and proceed with conducting the meeting in a more productive and relaxed manner. There are other impairments, namely cancer, multiple sclerosis, or any form of learning disability where there might be limitations in communication. Having a support person can help with such issues as they can act as a mediator between the person and their employer. Similarly, a support person can assist the employee in following a conversation, help them remember the concern that is being addressed, or take notes of the meeting.

Usually, a person whom the employee is familiar with can offer her or him moral support while attending an interview, an interactive accommodation meeting, a performance review meeting, or a disciplinary counseling.

HOW DOES AN EMPLOYER APPROVE FOR AN ACCOMMODATION?

In situations where an employee feels that she or he would be in a better position with the help of a support person, then the employer in all their power has to accommodate this. The employer may choose to question the employee to get an understanding of the requirements of the employee. This may include questions such as whether the employer can be certain if there is no hindrance in the process flow while working with a support person, what is the role that the support person plays on behalf of the employee, and why a support person is needed. Once the employer has the required information, she or he can proceed with making a decision on whether or not include a support person.

When the Employer Agrees That a Support Person Can Be Present

When the employer approved for a support person to be present, they have the full right to dictate some rules about that person's role during the meeting or interview. It can be useful to have a written policy of guideline so that all the parties involved in the meeting could understand her or his role in it to avoid disagreements or any other problems. The usual process of a meeting where a support person is present is that the employer follows the normal protocol that of any other meeting, and the support person acknowledges the guidelines of the process, knows and understands the employee by offering her or him their support when needed.

When the Employer Determines That a Support Person Is Not Required

In case the employer decides that a support person cannot be accommodated, then she or he is required to provide a valid reason for the rejection, give an explanation to the employee why she or he has arrived at that decision, and provide alternate solutions for the issue at hand. As per the employee's rights under the Americans with Disabilities Act (ADA), an employer cannot bluntly reject a support person as an accommodation. It would be considered a violation of rights and negatively contribute to disruption in the success and progress of the employee.

References
1. Whetzel, Melanie. "When Support Persons Hamper the Process They Were Brought In to Facilitate," Job Accommodation Network (JAN), n.d.
2. Whetzel, Melanie. "A Support Person as an Accommodation, Volume 05, Issue 01," Job Accommodation Network (JAN), November 19, 2010.
3. "Role of a Support Person," Queensland Government, July 31, 2020.

Section 49.4 | Addressing Stress-Related Concerns in the Workplace

This section contains text excerpted from the following sources: Text in this section begins with excerpts from "Mental Health in the Workplace," Centers for Disease Control and Prevention (CDC), April 10, 2019; Text beginning with the heading "What Is Job Stress" is excerpted from "Stress at Work," Centers for Disease Control and Prevention (CDC), February 1, 2001. Reviewed August 2020.

Mental-health disorders are among the most burdensome health concerns in the United States. Nearly 1 in 5 U.S. adults 18 years of age or older (18.3% or 44.7 million people) reported any mental illness in 2016. In addition, 71 percent of adults reported at least one symptom of stress, such as a headache or feeling overwhelmed or anxious.

Many people with mental-health disorders also need care for other physical-health conditions, including heart disease, diabetes, respiratory illness, and disorders that affect muscles, bones, and joints. The costs for treating people with both mental-health disorders and other physical conditions are 2 to 3 times higher than for those without co-occurring illnesses. By combining medical and behavioral-healthcare services, the United States could save $37.6 billion to $67.8 billion a year.

About 63 percent of Americans are part of the U.S. labor force. The workplace can be a key location for activities designed to improve well-being among adults. Workplace wellness programs can identify those at risk and connect them to treatment and put in place supports to help people reduce and manage stress. By addressing mental-health issues in the workplace, employers can reduce healthcare costs for their businesses and employees.

WHAT IS JOB STRESS?

Job stress can be defined as the harmful physical and emotional responses that occur when the requirements of the job do not match the capabilities, resources, or needs of the worker. Job stress can lead to poor health and even injury.

The concept of job stress is often confused with challenge, but these concepts are not the same. Challenge energizes us psychologically and physically, and it motivates us to learn new skills and master our jobs. When a challenge is met, we feel relaxed and satisfied. Thus, challenge is an important ingredient for healthy and productive work. The importance of challenge in our work lives is probably what people are referring to when they say "a little bit of stress is good for you."

JOB STRESS AND HEALTH

Stress sets off an alarm in the brain, which responds by preparing the body for defensive action. The nervous system is aroused and hormones are released to sharpen the senses, quicken the pulse, deepen respiration, and tense the muscles. This response (sometimes called the "fight" or "flight" response) is important because it helps us defend against threatening situations. The response is preprogrammed biologically. Everyone responds in much the same way, regardless of whether the stressful situation is at work or home.

Short-lived or infrequent episodes of stress pose little risk. But when stressful situations go unresolved, the body is kept in a constant state of activation, which increases the rate of wear and tear to biological systems. Ultimately, fatigue or damage results, and the ability of the body to repair and defend itself can become seriously compromised. As a result, the risk of injury or disease escalates.

In the past 20 years, many studies have looked at the relationship between job stress and a variety of ailments. Mood and sleep disturbances, upset stomach and headache, and disturbed relationships with family and friends are examples of stress-related problems that are quick to develop and are commonly seen in these studies. These early signs of job stress are usually easy to recognize. But, the effects of job stress on chronic diseases are more difficult to see because chronic diseases take a long time to develop and can be influenced by many factors other than stress. Nonetheless, evidence is rapidly accumulating to suggest that stress plays an important role in several types of chronic-health problems—especially cardiovascular disease (CVD), musculoskeletal disorders, and psychological disorders.

WHAT CAN BE DONE ABOUT JOB STRESS?

Stress management. Nearly one-half of large companies in the United States provide some type of stress management training for their workforces. Stress management programs teach workers about the nature and sources of stress, the effects of stress on health, and personal skills to reduce stress—for example, time management or relaxation exercises. (Employee assistance programs (EAPs) provide individual counseling for employees with both work and personal problems.) Stress management training may rapidly reduce stress symptoms such as anxiety and sleep disturbances; it also has the advantage of being inexpensive and easy to implement. However, stress management programs have two major disadvantages:

- The beneficial effects on stress symptoms are often short-lived.
- They often ignore important root causes of stress because they focus on the worker and not the environment.

371

Organizational change. This approach is the most direct way to reduce stress at work. It involves the identification of stressful aspects of work (e.g., excessive workload, conflicting expectations) and the design of strategies to reduce or eliminate the identified stressors. The advantage of this approach is that it deals directly with the root causes of stress at work. However, managers are sometimes uncomfortable with this approach because it can involve changes in work routines or production schedules, or changes in the organizational structure.

As a general rule, actions to reduce job stress should give top priority to organizational change to improve working conditions. But, even the most conscientious efforts to improve working conditions are unlikely to eliminate stress completely for all workers. For this reason, a combination of organizational change and stress management is often the most useful approach for preventing stress at work.

Chapter 50 | **Supporting a Person with an Anxiety Disorder**

Most people at some point in their lives, experience short periods of nervousness or anxiety, but this cannot be compared to what people with anxiety disorders go through everyday. Anxiety disorders make people feel shame, guilt, worry, and panic in situations where others do not experience such intense feelings. Anxiety affects not only the people who experience it, but it can also impact their loved ones, and it can be mentally demanding on both ends. This is because anxiety consumes people with an irrational fear of things that normal people can find hard to relate to.

HELPING A PERSON WITH ANXIETY

An anxious person is often completely overwhelmed by their anxiety, especially if they have a panic attack. This might make providing help and support intimidating and emotionally taxing. Sometimes, the symptoms of anxiety may not be diagnosed or they may be associated with stressful events in life, hormones, or considered a personality trait.

The following are some helpful suggestions to support a person with anxiety disorder:

Provide Validation and Concern

It is important to focus on the symptoms and patterns of anxiety in a person because each person experiences a different set of signs. One must learn to recognize the signs and triggers of anxiety and panic to be able to help a person avoid feelings of anxiousness or panic attacks. These are some common ways you can use to support a person with anxiety:

- Understand them and be supportive by listening and helping them work through their anxiety. Even if they do not wish to talk much about it, having someone who is trying to understand will be seen as helpful.
- When offering advice or helping them look at their fears from a rational perspective, try to be sympathetic to their feelings.
- Take efforts to consider their feelings of anxiety as an actual mental-health problem, and do not brush them away as pointless worry or making a scene.
- Ask them to seek help for their condition from a therapist or support their decision to get treated. You can also offer to secure appointments and make time to support them while they visit the doctor/therapist.

Help Identify and Break Free of Avoidance Behavior

A vital part of the development of anxiety disorders is avoidance behavior. When a person with anxiety avoids situations that cause anxiety, their feelings of anxiety will increase over time. Certain circumstances that incite avoidance behavior include:

- Making a phone call
- Getting started on an intimidating task, ranging from writing an essay to finishing up an annual work review
- Making requests, such as asking the boss for time off work

It is necessary to help a person identify and break free of avoidance behavior so they do not experience intrusive thoughts more often. You can help them take the first step in facing their fears and talk them through it to help them subdue their anxiety during stressful situations.

Do Not Enable Anxiety or Force Confrontation

When someone wishes to help their loved ones avoid things that cause feelings of panic and anxiety, it may seem understandable. However, this does not help a person with anxiety disorder, and constantly avoiding tough situations will enable their anxiety to grow even further. If you continue to adjust your behavior and the surroundings to accommodate a loved one's anxiety, it deprives them of the opportunity to get over their anxiety and face their problems.

Sometimes excessive anxiety can lead to severe depression, and they might need more help getting things done. In less extreme cases, you can offer little support without completely taking over or providing too much reassurance. At the same time, it is not alright to force someone into doing the things that make them anxious and panic. It is better to confer with a therapist to determine which situations to face and how to overcome them. It is beneficial to the patient to gain control over difficult situations one step at a time with guidance from an expert.

Destigmatize the Feeling of Anxiety

It is quite common for people to not discuss their mental-health problems with friends and family due to feelings of embarrassment. Stigma about mental health often exists due to misconceptions and lack of knowledge on the subject. People with anxiety fear their symptoms will show during a performance or in a social situation. For instance, they may be afraid of their voice shaking during a client meeting. It is important to come up with helpful strategies and reassure them that they can cope with such symptoms when or if they do occur.

You have to make them understand that their anxiety is not a weakness or a sign of incompetence. Normalize any anxious thoughts you can relate to, such as worrying about being judged and scared to ask for something due to fear of rejection. It is also common for people to have momentary thoughts about doing something weird or dangerous. For example, thinking about running over a pedestrian or the sudden urge to act violently. A person with anxiety disorder often does not realize that most people have such thoughts, and they constantly worry that they might act on one such fleeting thought.

EMERGENCY CRISIS

In some cases, when a person experiences severe anxiety or if their condition deteriorates rapidly, there is a possibility they may self-harm or attempt suicide. It is crucial to be prepared for such situations beforehand by talking to a person with an anxiety disorder when they are not experiencing a breakdown. A safety plan can be developed early on to cope if they are triggered and start getting suicidal thoughts.

PROBLEMS FACED BY CAREGIVERS

Given below are a few expected reactions when supporting a person with anxiety:

- **Denial.** When a person perceives their friend's anxiety is out of proportion to the minor issue at hand, they may have difficulty understanding and may end up disregarding their symptoms. For instance, telling them to get over it because it is all in their head.
- **Frustration.** This can happen when you have tried many strategies, but the person still feels worried and anxious.
- **Anxiousness.** Caring for a person with severe anxiety or panic attacks can sometimes affect you and create contagious feelings of anxiety.
- **Compassion fatigue.** This is caused by emotional and physical stress due to continually dealing with the anxious person's demands, which results in less ability to feel empathy towards them.

Often, it can be challenging and overwhelming to support a person with a mental-health condition. It is essential to take care of yourself, so you have the energy and time to help your loved one. Know your limits and set boundaries to support them as much as you possibly can without harming your mental health in the process. The caregiver's role can also be shared with others since it is easier to support someone if you share the responsibility.

References

1. "Self-care and Helping Someone with an Anxiety Disorder," The Royal Australian and New Zealand College of Psychiatrists, April 26, 2017.
2. "Caring for a Person Experiencing an Anxiety Disorder," Queensland Health, October 29, 2008.
3. Boyes, Alice. "Seven Ways to Help Someone with Anxiety," The Greater Good Science Center, July 25, 2018.
4. Boyes, Alice. "How to Help Someone With Anxiety," July 13, 2016.
5. "Anxiety and Panic Attacks," Mind, September 19, 2017.

Part 7 | Research on Anxiety Disorders

Chapter 51 | Role of Research in Improving the Understanding and Treatment of Anxiety Disorders

The mission of the National Institute of Mental Health (NIMH) is to reduce the burden of mental illness and behavioral disorders on the people of the United States through research on mind, brain, and behavior. An important corollary of this mission is to improve the treatment of these disorders. A critical activity in accomplishing this mission is developing and optimizing the use of treatments for mental illnesses in the United States. The NIMH, through the Division of Services and Intervention Research (DSIR), funds well over 100 treatment studies, many involving multiple sites, addressing important clinical questions that go beyond the scope and mission of the clinical trials conducted by the pharmaceutical industry in the private sector. These clinical trials are funded largely through investigator-initiated grants, but also through cooperative agreements and research contracts. In addition, training grants

This chapter contains text excerpted from the following sources: Text in this chapter begins with excerpts from "Treatment Research in Mental Illness: Improving the Nation's Public Mental Healthcare through NIMH Funded Interventions Research," National Institute of Mental Health (NIMH), January 2005. Reviewed August 2020; Text under the heading "Fast-Fail Trial Shows New Approach to Identifying Brain Targets for Clinical Treatments" is excerpted from "Fast-Fail Trial Shows New Approach to Identifying Brain Targets for Clinical Treatments," National Institute of Mental Health (NIMH), March 30, 2020.

support the career development of aspiring investigators in clinical treatment research. The scope of these trials covers all of the disorders in the NIMH purview, across the entire lifespan, including a diverse set of populations and employing an array of research designs and methodologies for studies of proof of concept, evaluation of efficacy/safety, and treatment effectiveness.

CREATING THE OPTIMAL TREATMENT RESEARCH PORTFOLIO

Treatment research in mental illness has some inherent differences from other forms of biomedical research and entails some unique challenges that must be overcome. Moreover, treatment research conducted by the pharmaceutical industry typically differs in fundamental ways from the kinds of studies that are required to inform mental-healthcare providers, administrators, and policy makers. Finally, to answer many questions in the treatment of mental illness, studies of great complexity and scale are required that often exceed the capacities of any one investigator or institution to conceive and orchestrate individually. The NIMH has already launched an effort to answer important clinical therapeutic issues through the funding of large clinical trials under the contract mechanism. However, the NIMH should adopt a more proactive strategy to further develop its treatment research programs and ensure that the most important clinical therapeutic and public mental-health issues are addressed in a methodologically rigorous and ecologically informative manner.

FAST-FAIL TRIAL SHOWS NEW APPROACH TO IDENTIFYING BRAIN TARGETS FOR CLINICAL TREATMENTS

A first-of-its-kind trial has demonstrated that a receptor involved in the brain's reward system may be a viable target for treating anhedonia (or lack of pleasure), a key symptom of several mood and anxiety disorders. This innovative fast-fail trial was funded by the NIMH, part of the NIH, and the results of the trial are published in *Nature Medicine.*

Mood and anxiety disorders are some of the most commonly diagnosed mental disorders, affecting millions of people each year. Despite this, available medications are not always effective in treating these disorders. The need for new treatments is clear, but developing psychiatric medications is often a resource-intensive process with a low success rate. To address this, NIMH established the Fast-Fail Trials program with the goal of enhancing the early phases of drug development.

"The fast-fail approach aims to help researchers determine—quickly and efficiently—whether targeting a specific neurobiological mechanism has the hypothesized effect and is a potential candidate for further clinical trials," explained Joshua A. Gordon, M.D., Ph.D., director of NIMH. "Positive results suggest that targeting a neurobiological mechanism affects brain function as expected, while negative results allow researchers to eliminate that target from further consideration. We hope this approach will pave the way towards the development of new and better treatments for individuals with mental illnesses."

Chapter 52 | **Research Studies on Behavioral Inhibition**

WHICH NEURONS ARE RESPONSIBLE FOR ANXIETY-RELATED BEHAVIORS?

Most people experience anxiety at some point in their lives, whether it is prespeech jitters or sweaty palms when their plane takes off. While mild feelings of nervousness are completely normal and can even be beneficial, anxiety can also have negative repercussions if it causes somebody to completely avoid situations like social encounters or taking a flight to visit distant family.

In a series of experiments, Intramural Research Program (IRP) researchers identified a specific set of neurons that appear to underlie certain fear-related avoidance behaviors in mice, potentially representing a useful target for treating human anxiety disorders.

Although mice enjoy surveying their surroundings, their position as the lowest link on the food chain makes them averse to brightly lit, open spaces where they might be snatched up by a hungry hawk. The way mice balance the risks and rewards of exploration mirrors many situations that can make humans anxious, says IRP investigator Alexxai V. Kravitz, Ph.D., the study's senior author.

"If you're buying a house, you're going to have a lot of excitement, but once the time to sign the contract comes, you're going

This chapter contains text excerpted from the following sources: Text under the heading "Which Neurons Are Responsible for Anxiety-Related Behaviors?" is excerpted from "Which Neurons Are Responsible for Anxiety-Related Behaviors?" National Institutes of Health (NIH), May 8, 2018; Text under the heading "Infant Temperament Predicts Introversion in Adulthood" is excerpted from "Infant Temperament Predicts Introversion in Adulthood," National Institutes of Health (NIH), April 28, 2020.

to think about the risks you're taking and whether this is the right decision," Dr. Kravitz explains. In other words, if signing makes you too nervous, you might just scrap the whole deal.

Past studies have suggested neurons that receive signals via the chemical dopamine in a brain area called the "striatum" are involved in assessing risk and reward and play a role in avoidance behaviors, as well as social phobia and some anxiety disorders. In the current study, IRP scientists led by first author Kimberly LeBlanc, Ph.D., a postdoctoral fellow in Dr. Kravitz's lab, first examined the behavior of mice that did not have a specific dopamine receptor, the dopamine D2 receptor, in those striatal neurons. Since dopamine receptors convert dopamine-based signals into usable messages, this lack of dopamine receptors made the neurons less sensitive to dopamine-based communication.

Compared to control mice with intact D2 receptors throughout their brains, mice that lacked the D2 receptor in striatal cells called "indirect medium spiny neurons" (iMSNs) spent less time in open spaces during behavioral tests that allowed them to freely move between enclosed and open areas. Importantly, these behavioral changes were independent of overall changes in the animals' movements, so the mice did not stay in the enclosed areas simply because they were moving around less. Mice missing the D2 receptor in other populations of neurons did not differ from the control mice, suggesting D2 receptors specifically in the iMSNs are important for avoidance behaviors in mice.

"Knocking out this receptor alters the timing of these neurons' activity," Dr. Kravitz explains. "Normally, the activity of all the neurons in the brain is very precisely timed, like a piece of music, and it produces this very nice synchronized behavior. If the timing of this activity is altered—like, say, one neuron fires a second too early and another one a second too late—the animal gets stuck in a state where it is not executing these exploratory movements."

Similarly, when Dr. Kravitz's team directly disrupted the timing of iMSN activity in genetically normal mice, the animals became more risk averse and spent less time in open spaces. On the other hand, when the scientists inhibited those neurons, the mice spent more time in the exposed areas.

"Knowing that this cell type is important for anxiety-related behaviors, you can drill down and ask how you can gain pharmacological access to this system," Dr. Kravitz says. "Is there a drug that would preferentially act on these neurons?"

However, because there are so many varieties of anxiety disorders, Dr. Kravitz cautions that designing treatments to tamp down the activity of those cells may not be a panacea.

"Anxiety disorders are incredibly hard to treat because there's not just one problem where everyone can have the same treatment," he explains, "so even if this work is successful, it might help only a subset of people with severe anxiety."

INFANT TEMPERAMENT PREDICTS INTROVERSION IN ADULTHOOD

We each have different temperaments that are fairly stable over time. Temperament is the biologically based way a person tends to emotionally and behaviorally respond to the world. Temperament during infancy can serve as the foundation for personality over time. One type of temperament, called "behavioral inhibition," is characterized by cautious, fearful behavior toward unfamiliar people, objects, and situations. Behavioral inhibition is relatively stable across toddlerhood and childhood. Children with behavioral inhibition are at elevated risk for developing so-called internalizing conditions such as social withdrawal and anxiety disorders. The brain's error monitoring system is thought to play a role in such conditions. This can be seen on electroencephalogram (EEG) brain recordings. Negative dips show up when a person makes an error on a computerized task. This is called "error-related negativity," (ERN). ERN reflects how sensitive a person is to their errors. A larger ERN has been associated with behavioral inhibition, while a smaller ERN has been linked with conditions such as impulsivity and substance use.

To investigate whether behavioral inhibition in infancy can predict personality traits in adulthood, a research team led by Drs. Daniel Pine at National Institutes of Health's (NIH) National Institute of Mental Health (NIMH) and Nathan Fox at the University of Maryland recruited 165 infants at 4 months of age and assessed them for behavioral inhibition based on observation at 14 months.

When the infants were 15 years of age, the researchers recorded ERN on EEGs. The participants then returned at age 26 for assessments of psychopathology, personality, social functioning, and education and employment outcomes.

The team found that behavioral inhibition at 14 months of age predicted, by age 26, a more reserved personality, fewer romantic relationships, and lower social functioning with friends and family. It also predicted higher levels of internalizing behaviors in adulthood, particularly among those who also displayed larger ERN signals at age 15. Behavioral inhibition was not associated with education and employment outcomes.

"We have studied the biology of behavioral inhibition over time, and it is clear that it has a profound effect influencing developmental outcome," Fox says.

Chapter 53 | Pediatrics-Based Brief Therapy Outdoes Referral for Youths with Anxiety and Depression

A streamlined behavioral therapy delivered in a pediatrics practice offered much greater benefit to youth with anxiety and depression than a more standard referral to mental healthcare with follow-up in a clinical trial comparing the two approaches. The benefit of the former approach in comparison with referral was especially striking in Hispanic youth, a finding that may help inform efforts to address disparities in care.

Depression and anxiety disorders are prevalent among youth; an estimated 25.1 percent of 13 to 18-year-olds have an anxiety disorder. Surveys also suggest that less than a third of youth with anxiety and just over 40 percent with mood disorders receive treatment. These disorders can have serious consequences for affected youth; depression and anxiety can compromise education, employment, and relationships with friends and family.

V. Robin Weersing, Ph.D., at San Diego State University, and David A. Brent, M.D., at the University of Pittsburgh, led the clinical trial, which enrolled 185 youths, 8 to 16 years of age, from

This chapter includes text excerpted from "Pediatrics-Based Brief Therapy Outdoes Referral for Youths with Anxiety and Depression," National Institute of Mental Health (NIMH), May 31, 2017.

pediatric clinics in San Diego and Pittsburgh. Participants in the trial met criteria for depression or an anxiety disorder, including separation anxiety, generalized anxiety disorder (GAD), or social phobia. Each was randomly assigned to either a brief behavioral therapy (BBT) or to referral to mental healthcare with periodic check-in calls ("assisted referral").

The BBT tested in this trial simultaneously addresses both depression and anxiety, rather than targeting one or the other, and it is streamlined in comparison to some standard approaches, with fewer therapeutic components. Of the 95 youths assigned to BBT in the trial, 50 (56.8%) improved on a scale that assesses improvement across anxiety and depression, while 20 (28.2%) of youths in the assisted referral group improved. Raters who evaluated the youth were unaware of which treatment each received. Youth in the BBT group also did better on a scale of overall functioning and had fewer symptoms of anxiety.

The contrast in results between the Hispanic youth receiving BBT and those receiving assisted referral was even greater: 13 of 17 (76.5%) responded to BBT, while 1 of 14 (7.1%) assigned to assisted referral did. Hispanic youths receiving BBT also did much better on measures of functioning.

One of the central elements of the BBT was behavioral activation in which a youth is encouraged to engage in activities that she or he finds desirable but difficult, such as social functions. "In these interventions, kids learn not to withdraw from what is upsetting them," said Dr. Weersing, lead author and developer of the intervention. "Slowly they learn to approach and actively problem solve. Step by step, they re-engage with the tasks that they need to do or want to do—school, social, family-related—but previously struggled to do, because negative emotions were in the way."

Any differences in the number of therapeutic sessions received either with BBT or as a result of referral did not account for the differences measured in benefits to youth. The referral coordinators successfully connected 82 percent of families with specialty mental healthcare, and the youth in that group had an average of 6.5 therapeutic visits (versus an average of 11.2 sessions of BBT). But, even the referral group youth with the most therapeutic sessions had worse outcomes than those in BBT.

Pediatrics-Based Brief Therapy

An important impetus for the development of the therapy tested in this trial was to provide an intervention that is easy to disseminate, and in particular, adaptable for use in primary care settings where many children and adolescents get regular care. "In order to reach the very large number of youth suffering from emotional problems, we need to explore treatment delivery settings, like pediatrics, with a wide reach and low stigma," said Dr. Weersing. "This has great promise for improving access to care, particularly for Latinx youth."

Chapter 54 | Circuitry for Fearful Feelings, Behavior Untangled in Anxiety Disorders

An "incorrect" assumption that fear and anxiety are mediated in the brain by a single "fear circuit" has stalled progress in developing better treatments for anxiety disorders, argue two leading experts. Designing future research based on a "two-system" framework holds promise for improving treatment outcomes, say Daniel Pine, M.D., a clinical researcher in the National Institute of Mental Health (NIMH) Emotion and Development Branch, and Joseph LeDoux, Ph.D., a basic scientist and NIMH grantee at New York University.

Neuroscience advances in understanding how the brain detects and responds to threat have failed to translate into significantly improved treatments because the field has been led astray by a simplistic notion of a "fear system," contend Pine and LeDoux. For example, hopes that medications that lessen rodents' stress reactivity might help people feel less fearful or anxious often have not borne out.

This chapter contains text excerpted from the following sources: Text under the heading "Circuitry for Fearful Feelings, Behavior Untangled in Anxiety Disorders" is excerpted from "Circuitry for Fearful Feelings, Behavior Untangled in Anxiety Disorders," National Institute of Mental Health (NIMH), September 9, 2016. Reviewed August 2020; Text under the heading "Researchers Identify Key Brain Circuits for Reward-Seeking and Avoidance Behavior" is excerpted from "Researchers Identify Key Brain Circuits for Reward-Seeking and Avoidance Behavior," National Institute of Mental Health (NIMH), August 22, 2018.

Rather, the authors point to mounting evidence that such subjective feeling states are mediated via different circuitry than defensive behaviors. The former via higher order processing in the cortex—and the latter via the amygdala and related centers, mostly deeper in the brain.

For starters, Pine and LeDoux propose more precise use of terminology. Fear and anxiety describe conscious subjective feeling states; defensive reactions refer to rapidly-deployed behaviors or physiological responses. Fear denotes feelings associated with an imminent threat, anxiety feelings associated with an uncertain or more distant source of harm.

For example, the amygdala, often colloquially dubbed the brain's "fear center," in fact unconsciously detects and responds to imminent threats and contributes to fear only indirectly. States such as fear and anxiety instead arise from areas of the cortex associated with higher order thinking processes and language in people, only some of which occur in other animals.

"If feelings of fear or anxiety are not products of circuits that control defensive behavior, studies of defensive behavior in animals will be of limited value in finding medications that can relieve feelings of fear and anxiety in people," observe the authors, who note that making such distinctions will help in the design of more realistic translational studies.

Meanwhile, the distinctions may also temper expectations for development of specific-acting antianxiety agents. "Existing medications are blunt tools," note Pine and LeDoux. If the experience of fear and anxiety is rooted in cortical changes in thinking, attention and memory, some "anxiolytic" effects might result from "general emotional blunting" or "impaired cognitive processing," they add.

Improving treatments will require a more exact understanding of how treatments work. With this knowledge and the two-systems perspective, existing treatments might be adapted to work better. Brain imaging biomarkers might help tailor treatments to target circuit dysfunctions of specific patients. For example, anxious patients showing altered activity profiles in cortex circuitry underlying working memory might receive psychotherapies that teach them how to regulate emotion through reappraisal or other thinking strategies.

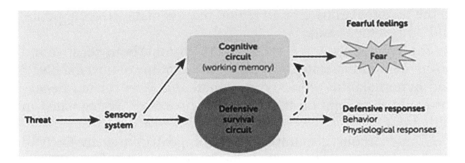

Figure 54.1. The Two-System Model

RESEARCHERS IDENTIFY KEY BRAIN CIRCUITS FOR REWARD-SEEKING AND AVOIDANCE BEHAVIOR

Researchers have identified connections between neurons in brain systems associated with reward, stress, and emotion. Conducted in mice, the new study may help untangle multiple psychiatric conditions, including alcohol-use disorder, anxiety disorders, insomnia, and depression in humans.

"Understanding these intricate brain systems will be critical for developing diagnostic and therapeutic tools for a broad array of conditions," said George F. Koob, Ph.D., director of the National Institute on Alcohol Abuse and Alcoholism (NIAAA), which contributed funding for the study. The NIMH also provided major support for the research. The NIAAA and NIMH are parts of the National Institutes of Health (NIH).

Responding appropriately to aversive or rewarding stimuli is essential for survival. This requires fine-tuned regulation of brain systems that enable rapid responses to changes in the environment, such as those involved in sleep, wakefulness, stress, and reward-seeking. These same brain systems are often dysregulated in addiction and other psychiatric conditions.

In the new study, researchers looked at the extended amygdala, a brain region involved in fear, arousal, and emotional processing and which plays a significant role in drug and alcohol addiction. They focused on a part of this structure known as the "bed nucleus of stria terminalis" (BNST), which connects the extended amygdala to the hypothalamus, a brain region that regulates sleep, appetite, and body temperature.

The hypothalamus is also thought to promote both negative and positive emotional states. A better understanding of how the BNST and hypothalamus work to coordinate emotion-related behavior could shed light on the emotional processes dysregulated in addiction.

"These circuits, also implicated in binge drinking, are likely to be elements in understanding the detailed mechanisms driving stress-related alcohol- or drug-seeking and consummatory behaviors," said first author Dr. Giardino.

To map the brain circuitry between the BNST and the hypothalamus, Dr. Giardino and his colleagues exposed mice to rewarding and aversive stimuli, and then visualized and manipulated the activity of neurons using fiber optic techniques.

The scientists identified two distinct subpopulations of neurons in the BNST that connect to separate populations of neurons in the lateral hypothalamus. These parallel circuits drove opposing emotional states: avoidance (aversion) and approach (preference). Different neurotransmitters were linked to aversion and preference within these neurocircuits—corticotropin releasing factor was involved in aversion, while cholecystokinin played a role in preference.

Chapter 55 | Brain Imaging for Mental Disorders

BRAIN RESEARCH

Modern research tools and techniques are giving scientists a more detailed understanding of the brain than ever before.

Brain Imaging

Using brain imaging technologies, such as magnetic resonance imaging (MRI), which uses magnetic fields to take pictures of the brain's structure, studies show that brain growth in children with autism appears to peak early. And as they grow there are differences in brain development in children who develop bipolar disorder than children who do not.

Studies comparing such children to those with normal brain development may help scientists to pinpoint when and where mental disorders begin and perhaps how to slow or stop them from progressing. Functional magnetic resonance imaging (fMRI) is another important research tool in understanding how the brain functions.

Another type of brain scan called "magnetoencephalography," or "MEG," can capture split-second changes in the brain. Using MEG, some scientists have found a specific pattern of brain activity that may help predict who is most likely to respond to fast-acting antidepressant medications. Currently available antidepressants usually

This chapter contains text excerpted from the following sources: Text under the heading "Brain Research" is excerpted from "Introduction: Brain Basics," National Institute of Mental Health (NIMH), July 5, 2016. Reviewed August 2020; Text under the heading "Mental Illness Defined as Disruption in Neural Circuits" is excerpted from "Post by Former NIMH Director Thomas Insel: Mental Illness Defined as Disruption in Neural Circuits," National Heart, Lung, and Blood Institute (NHLBI), August 12, 2011. Reviewed August 2020.

take four to six weeks to reach their full effect, which can be a difficult wait for some people struggling with depression. However, recent research points to a possible new class of antidepressants that can relieve symptoms of the illness in just a few hours. Knowing who might respond to such medications could reduce the amount of trial and error and frustration that many people with depression experience when starting treatment.

Gene Studies

Advanced technologies are also making it faster, easier, and more affordable to study genes. Scientists have found many different genes and groups of genes that appear to increase risk or provide protection from various mental disorders. Other genes may change the way a person responds to a certain medication. This information may someday make it possible to predict who will develop a mental disorder and to tailor the treatment for a person's specific conditions.

Such brain research helps increase the understanding of how the brain grows and works and the effects of genes and environment on mental health. This knowledge is allowing scientists to make important discoveries that could change the way we think about and treat mental illnesses.

MENTAL ILLNESS DEFINED AS DISRUPTION IN NEURAL CIRCUITS

It has become an NIMH mantra to describe mental disorders as brain disorders. What does this mean? Is it accurate to group schizophrenia, depression, and ADHD together with Alzheimer disease (AD), Parkinson disease (PD), and Huntington disease? Is a neurologic approach to mental disorders helpful or does this focus on the brain lead to less attention to the mind?

First, mental disorders appear to be disorders of brain circuits, in contrast to classical neurological disorders in which focal lesions are apparent. By analogy, heart disease can involve arrhythmias or infarction (death) of heart muscle. Both can be fatal, but the arrhythmia may not have a demonstrable lesion. In past decades, there was little hope of finding abnormal brain circuitry beyond the coarse approach of an electroencephalogram (EEG), which revealed little detail about regional cortical function. With the advent of imaging techniques such as positron emission tomography (PET), functional magnetic resonance imaging (fMRI), magnetoencephalography (MEG), and high resolution EEG, the broad range of cortical function with high spatial and temporal resolution can be mapped. For the first time, the mind via the brain can be studied. Mapping patterns of cortical activity reveals mechanisms of mental function that are just not apparent by observing behavior.

Has brain imaging been useful for understanding mental disorders? While we are still in the early days of using these powerful technologies, a recent survey of the literature reveals some excellent examples of how studying the brain forces us to "rethink" mental disorders. For instance, studies of brain development demonstrate delays in cortical maturation in children with ADHD. How curious that this disorder, which is defined by cognitive (attention) and behavioral (hyperactivity) symptoms, increasingly appears to be a disorder of cortical development. Viewing ADHD as a brain disorder raises new, important questions: What does cause delayed maturation? What treatments might accelerate cortical development?

A brain disorder approach also may transform the way the mental disorders are diagnosed. The NIMH Research Domain Criteria (R-DoC) project is involved in rethinking diagnosis based on understanding the underlying brain changes. As an example, what is now called as "major depressive disorder" probably represents many unique syndromes, responding to different interventions. Neuroimaging is beginning to yield biomarkers, that is, patterns that predict response to treatment or possibly reflect changes in physiology prior to changes in behavior or mood. And studies with deep brain stimulation addressing depression as a "brain arrhythmia" are demonstrating how changing the activity of specific circuits leads to remission of otherwise treatment refractory depressive episodes.

An important implication of this new approach is that abnormal behavior and cognition (e.g., mood, attention) may be late and convergent outcomes of altered brain development. This is a familiar lesson from neurodegenerative disorders: the symptoms of Alzheimer, Parkinson, and Huntington diseases emerge years after changes in the brain. Could the same be true of these circuit disorders that appear early in life? If so, could imaging allow earlier detection and preemption of the behavioral and cognitive changes—from the social isolation of autism to the psychosis of schizophrenia? This preemptive approach, which has transformed outcomes in heart disease and cancer, could also transform psychiatry, by focusing on prevention for those at risk rather than the partial amelioration of symptoms late in the process.

But, there is a need to recognize the range of unknowns that remain. In truth, we still do not know how to define a circuit. Where does a circuit begin or end? How do the patterns of "activity" on imaging scans actually translate to what is happening in the brain? What is the direction of information flow? In fact, the metaphor of a circuit in the sense of flow of electricity may be woefully inadequate for describing how mental activity emerges from neuronal activity in the brain. Hence, the need for continuing research into fundamental neuroscience. The advent of new tools, such as optogenetics, which uses light for precise manipulation of cells in awake, behaving animals will take us a long way towards understanding the characteristics of a neuronal circuit.

While the neuroscience discoveries are coming fast and furious, one thing that can be said already is that earlier notions of mental disorders as chemical imbalances or as social constructs are beginning to look antiquated. Much of what we are learning about the neural basis of mental illness is not yet ready for the clinic, but there can be little doubt that clinical neuroscience will soon be helping people with mental disorders to recover.

Part 8 | Additional Help and Information

Chapter 56 | Glossary of Terms Related to Anxiety Disorders

abandonment: A situation in which the child has been left by the parent(s), the parent's identity or whereabouts are unknown.

acupuncture: A family of procedures involving stimulation of anatomical points on the body by a variety of techniques.

addiction: A chronic, relapsing disease characterized by compulsive seeking and use of any addictive agent and by long-lasting changes in the brain.

adolescence: A human life stage that begins at twelve years of age and continues until twenty-one complete years of age, generally marked by the beginning of puberty and lasting to the beginning of adulthood.

agitation: A condition in which a person is unable to relax and be still. The person may be very tense and irritable, and become easily annoyed by small things.

agoraphobia: An intense fear of being in open places or in situations where it may be hard to escape, or where help may not be available.

amygdala: An almond-shaped structure involved in processing and remembering strong emotions such as fear. It is part of the limbic system and located deep inside the brain.

anorexia nervosa: An eating disorder caused by a person having a distorted body image and not consuming the appropriate calorie intake resulting in severe weight loss.

antidepressant: Medication used to treat depression and other mood and anxiety disorders.

This glossary contains terms excerpted from documents produced by several sources deemed reliable.

anxiety: An abnormal sense of fear, nervousness, and apprehension about something that might happen in the future.

avoidance: One of the symptoms of posttraumatic stress disorder (PTSD). Those with PTSD avoid situations and reminders of their trauma.

behavior problem: Behavior of the child in the school and/or community that adversely affects socialization, learning, growth, and moral development. May include adjudicated or nonadjudicated behavior problems. Includes running away from home or a placement.

behavioral health: A state of mental/emotional being and/or choices and actions that affect wellness. Substance abuse and misuse, as well as serious psychological distress, suicide, and mental illness, are examples of some behavioral-health problems.

behavioral therapy: Behavioral therapy focuses on a person's actions and aims to change unhealthy behavior patterns.

biofeedback: A technique that uses simple electronic devices to teach clients how to consciously regulate bodily functions, such as breathing, heart rate, and blood pressure, to improve overall health. Biofeedback is used to reduce stress, eliminate headaches, recondition injured muscles, control asthma attacks, and relieve pain.

bipolar disorder: A disorder that causes severe and unusually high and low shifts in mood, energy, and activity levels, as well as unusual shifts in the ability to carry out day-to-day tasks (also known as "manic depression").

bonding: The process of developing lasting emotional ties with one's immediate caregivers; seen as the first and primary developmental achievement of a human being and central to a person's ability to relate to others throughout life.

borderline personality disorder (BPD): BPD is a serious mental illness marked by unstable moods, behavior, and relationships.

cognition: Conscious mental activities (such as thinking, communicating, understanding, solving problems, processing information, and remembering) that are associated with gaining knowledge and understanding.

cognitive-behavioral therapy (CBT): CBT helps people focus on how to solve their current problems. The therapist helps the patient learn how to identify distorted or unhelpful thinking patterns, recognize and change inaccurate beliefs, relate to others in more positive ways, and change behaviors accordingly.

Glossary of Terms Related to Anxiety Disorders

comorbidity: The existence of two or more illnesses in the same person. These illnesses can be physical or mental.

deep breathing: An active process that involves conscious control over breathing in and out. This may involve controlling the way in which air is drawn in (e.g., through the mouth or nostrils), the rate (e.g., quickly or over a length of time), the depth (e.g., shallow or deep), and the control of other body parts (e.g., relaxation of the stomach).

depression: Lack of interest or pleasure in daily activities, sadness and feelings of worthlessness or excessive guilt that are severe enough to interfere with working, sleeping, studying, eating, and enjoying life.

discipline: Training that develops self-control, self-sufficiency, and orderly conduct. Discipline is based on respect for an individual's capability and is not to be confused with punishment.

dopamine: A brain chemical, classified as a neurotransmitter, found in regions of the brain that regulate movement, emotion, and motivation.

drug abuse: Compulsive use of drugs that is not of a temporary nature. Applies to infants addicted at birth.

early intervention: Diagnosing and treating a mental illness when it first develops.

eating disorder: Mental illnesses such as anorexia nervosa, bulimia nervosa, and binge eating disorder (BED), involve serious problems with eating.

gene: The basic unit of heredity, composed of a segment of DNA containing the code for a specific trait.

hallucinations: Hearing, seeing, touching, smelling, or tasting things that are not real.

hormone: A chemical message produced by an endocrine gland which travels through the bloodstream to a target organ.

hypnosis: An altered state of consciousness characterized by increased responsiveness to suggestion. The procedure is used to effect positive changes and to treat numerous health conditions including ulcers, chronic pain, respiratory ailments, stress, and headaches.

impulse: An electrical communication signal sent between neurons to communicate with each other.

insomnia: A chronic or acute sleep disorder characterized by a complaint of difficulty initiating, and/or maintaining sleep, and/or a subjective complaint of poor sleep quality.

isolation: State of being separated from others. Isolation is sometimes used to prevent disease from spreading.

massage therapy: This type of therapy encompasses many different techniques. In general, therapists press, rub, and otherwise manipulate the muscles and other soft tissues of the body.

meditation: A group of techniques, most of which started in Eastern religious or spiritual traditions. In meditation, individuals learn to focus their attention and suspend the stream of thoughts that normally occupy the mind. This practice is believed to result in a state of greater physical relaxation, mental calmness, and psychological balance. Practicing meditation can change how a person relates to the flow of emotions and thoughts in the mind.

mental illness: A health condition that changes a person's thinking, feelings, or behavior (or all three) and that causes the person distress and difficulty in functioning.

mood disorders: Mental disorders primarily affecting a person's mood.

obsessive-compulsive disorder (OCD): An anxiety disorder in which a person suffers from obsessive thoughts and compulsive actions such as cleaning, checking, counting, or hoarding.

panic disorder (PD): An anxiety disorder in which a person suffers from sudden attacks of fear and panic. The attacks may occur without a known reason, but many times they are triggered by events or thoughts that produce fear in the person, such as taking an elevator or driving.

phobia: An anxiety disorder in which a person suffers from an unusual amount of fear of a certain activity or situation.

postpartum depression: A mental-health condition when a new mother has a major depressive episode within one month after delivery.

posttraumatic stress disorder (PTSD): An anxiety disorder that develops in reaction to physical injury or severe mental or emotional distress such as military combat, violent assault, natural disaster, or other life-threatening events.

psychiatrist: A doctor (M.D.) who treats mental illness. Psychiatrists must receive additional training and serve a supervised residency in their specialty. They can prescribe medications.

psychologist: A clinical psychologist is a professional who treats mental illness, emotional disturbance, and behavior problems. They use talk therapy as treatment, and cannot prescribe medication. A clinical psychologist will have a master's degree (M.A.) or doctorate (Ph.D.) in psychology, and possibly more training in a specific type of therapy.

psychosis: The word "psychosis" is used to describe conditions that affect the mind, where there has been some loss of contact with reality (delusions and hallucinations). When someone becomes ill in this way it is called a "psychotic episode." During a period of psychosis, a person's thoughts and perceptions are disturbed and the individual may have difficulty understanding what is real and what is not.

schizophrenia: A severe mental disorder that appears in late adolescence or early adulthood. People with schizophrenia may have hallucinations, delusions, loss of personality, confusion, agitation, social withdrawal, psychosis, and/or extremely odd behavior.

sedative: Drugs that suppress anxiety and promote sleep; the National Survey on Drug Use and Health (NSDUH) classification includes benzodiazepines, barbiturates, and other types of CNS depressants.

selective serotonin reuptake inhibitors (SSRIs): A group of medications used to treat depression. These medications cause an increase in the amount of the neurotransmitter serotonin in the brain.

serotonin: A neurotransmitter present throughout the body and brain that plays an important role in headache and migraine, mood disorders, regulating body temperature, sleep, vomiting, sexuality, and appetite.

sexual abuse: Coercing or attempting to coerce any sexual contact or behavior without consent

social phobia: It is a strong fear of being judged by others and of being embarrassed. This fear can be so strong that it gets in the way of going to work or school or doing other everyday things.

tai chi: A mind-body practice that originated in China as a martial art. Individuals doing tai chi move their bodies slowly and gently, while breathing deeply and meditating. (Tai chi is sometimes called "moving meditation.")

traumatic event: An event, or series of events, that causes moderate-to-severe stress reactions, is called a "traumatic event." Traumatic events are characterized by a sense of horror, helplessness, serious injury, or the threat of serious injury or death.

yoga: A combination of breathing exercises, physical postures, and meditation used to calm the nervous system and balance the body, mind, and spirit.

Chapter 57 | Directory of Organizations That Help People with Anxiety Disorders and Other Mental-Health Concerns

GOVERNMENT ORGANIZATIONS

Agency for Healthcare Research and Quality (AHRQ)
Office of Communications
5600 Fishers Ln.
Seventh Fl.
Rockville, MD 20857
Phone: 301-427-1104
Website: www.ahrq.gov

Center for Mental Health Services (CMHS)
Substance Abuse and Mental
Health Services Administration
(SAMHSA)
5600 Fishers Ln.
Rockville, MD 20857
Phone: 240-276-1310
Website: www.samhsa.
gov/about-us/who-we-are/
offices-centers/cmhs

Resources in this chapter were compiled from several sources deemed reliable; all contact information was verified and updated in August 2020.

Centers for Disease Control and Prevention (CDC)
1600 Clifton Rd.
Atlanta, GA 30329-4027
Toll-Free: 800-CDC-INFO
(800-232-4636)
Phone: 404-639-3311
Toll-Free TTY: 888-232-6348
Website: www.cdc.gov
E-mail: cdcinfo@cdc.gov

Eunice Kennedy Shriver National Institute of Child Health and Human Development (NICHD)
NICHD Information Resource
Center (IRC)
P.O. Box 3006
Rockville, MD 20847
Toll-Free: 800-370-2943
Phone: 301-496-5133
Toll-Free Fax: 866-760-5947
Website: www.nichd.nih.gov
E-mail:
NICHDInformationResource
Center@mail.nih.gov

MedlinePlus
U.S. National Library of Medicine
(NLM)
8600 Rockville Pike
Bethesda, MD 20894
Toll-Free: 888-FIND-NLM
(888-346-3656)
Phone: 301-594-5983
Website: www.medlineplus.gov

National Center for Complementary and Integrative Health (NCCIH)
9000 Rockville Pike
Bethesda, MD 20892
Toll-Free: 888-644-6226
Toll-Free TTY: 866-464-3615
Website: nccih.nih.gov
E-mail: info@nccih.nih.gov

National Institute of Mental Health (NIMH)
Office of Science Policy, Planning,
and Communications (OSPPC)
6001 Executive Blvd.
Rm. 6200, MSC 9663
Bethesda, MD 20892-9663
Toll-Free: 866-615-NIMH
(866-615-6464)
Toll-Free TTY: 866-415-8051
Fax: 301-443-4279
Website: www.nimh.nih.gov
E-mail: nimhinfo@nih.gov

National Institute on Aging (NIA)
31 Center Dr., MSC 2292
Bldg. 31, Rm. 5C27
Bethesda, MD 20892
Toll-Free: 800-222-2225
Toll-Free TTY: 800-222-4225
Website: www.nia.nih.gov
E-mail: niaic@nia.nih.gov

National Institute on Alcohol Abuse and Alcoholism (NIAAA)

Toll-Free: 888-MY-NIAAA
(888-696-4222)
Phone: 301-443-3860
Website: www.niaaa.nih.gov
E-mail: niaaaweb-r@exchange.nih.gov

National Institute on Deafness and Other Communication Disorders (NIDCD)

31 Center Dr.
MSC 2320
Bethesda, MD 20892-2320
Fax: 301-402-0018
Website: www.nidcd.nih.gov
E-mail: nidcdinfo@nidcd.nih.gov

National Institute on Drug Abuse (NIDA)

Office of Science Policy and
Communications (OSPC)
6001 Executive Blvd.
Rm. 5213, MSC 9561
Bethesda, MD 20892
Phone: 301-443-1124
Website: www.drugabuse.gov

National Institutes of Health (NIH)

9000 Rockville Pike
Bethesda, MD 20892
Phone: 301-496-4000
Website: www.nih.gov

NIH News in Health

NIH Office of Communications
and Public Liaison (OCPL)
Bldg. 31, Rm. 5B52
Bethesda, MD 20892-2094
Phone: 301-451-8224
Website: newsinhealth.nih.gov
E-mail: nihnewsinhealth@od.nih.gov

Office on Women's Health (OWH)

U.S. Department of Health and
Human Services (HHS)
200 Independence Ave., S.W.
Rm. 712E
Washington, DC 20201
Toll-Free: 800-994-9662
Phone: 202-690-7650
Fax: 202-205-2631
Website: www.womenshealth.gov

Social Security Administration (SSA)

1100 W. High Rise
6401 Security Blvd.
Baltimore, MD 21235
Toll-Free: 800-772-1213
Toll-Free TTY: 800-325-0778
Website: www.ssa.gov

Substance Abuse and Mental Health Services Administration (SAMHSA)

5600 Fishers Ln.
Rockville, MD 20857
Toll-Free: 877-SAMHSA-7
(877-726-4727)
Toll-Free TTY: 800-487-4889
Website: www.samhsa.gov
E-mail: SAMHSAInfo@samhsa.hhs.gov

U.S. Department of Health and Human Services (HHS)
200 Independence Ave., S.W.
Washington, DC 20201
Toll-Free: 877-696-6775
Website: www.hhs.gov

U.S. Department of Labor (DOL)
200 Constitution Ave., N.W.
Washington, DC 20210
Toll-Free: 866-4-USA-DOL
(866-487-2365)
Website: www.dol.gov

U.S. Department of Veterans Affairs (VA)
Toll-Free: 844-698-2311
TTY: 711
Website: www.va.gov

U.S. Equal Employment Opportunity Commission (EEOC)
131 M St., N.E.
Fourth Fl., Ste. 4NWO2F
Washington, DC 20507-0100
Toll-Free: 800-669-4000
Phone: 202-663-4900
Toll-Free TTY: 800-669-6820
Fax: 202-419-0739
Website: www.eeoc.gov
E-mail: info@eeoc.gov

PRIVATE ORGANIZATIONS

Academy of Cognitive & Behavioral Therapies
Academy of Cognitive Therapy,
Department of Psychiatry
245 N. 15th St., MS 403
17 New College Bldg.
Philadelphia, PA 19102
Phone: 215-831-7838
Fax: 215-537-1789
Website: www.academyofct.org
E-mail: info@academyofct.org

Al-Anon Family Groups
1600 Corporate Landing Pkwy
Virginia Beach, VA 23454-5617
Phone: 757-563-1600
Fax: 757-563-1656
Website: al-anon.org
E-mail: wso@al-anon.org

American Academy of Child and Adolescent Psychiatry (AACAP)
3615 Wisconsin Ave., N.W.
Washington, DC 20016-3007
Phone: 202-966-7300
Fax: 202-464-0131
Website: www.aacap.org

American Association for Geriatric Psychiatry (AAGP)
6728 Old McLean Village Dr.
McLean, VA 22101
Phone: 703-556-9222
Fax: 703-556-8729
Website: www.aagponline.org

American Counseling Association (ACA)

6101 Stevenson Ave., Ste. 600
Alexandria, VA 22304
Toll-Free: 800-473-2329
Phone: 703-823-9800
Fax: 703-823-0252
Website: www.counseling.org

American Foundation for Suicide Prevention (AFSP)

199 Water St.
11th Fl.
New York, NY 10038
Toll-Free: 888-333-2377
Phone: 212-363-3500
Fax: 212-363-6237
Website: afsp.org
E-mail: info@afsp.org

American Group Psychotherapy Association (AGPA)

25 E. 21st St., Sixth Fl.
New York, NY 10010
Phone: 212-477-2677
Fax: 212-979-6627
Website: www.agpa.org
E-mal: info@agpa.org

American Psychiatric Association (APA)

800 Maine Ave., S.W.
Ste. 900
Washington, DC 20024
Toll-Free: 888-357-7924
(888-35-PSYCH)
Phone: 202-559-3900
Website: www.psychiatry.org
E-mail: apa@psych.org

American Psychological Association (APA)

750 First St. N.E.
Washington, DC 20002-4242
Toll-Free: 800-374-2721
Phone: 202-336-5500
TDD/TTY: 202-336-6123
Website: www.apa.org
E-mail: customerservice@apa.org

Association for Behavioral and Cognitive Therapies (ABCT)

305 7th Ave.
16th Fl.
New York, NY 10001
Phone: 212-647-1890
Fax: 212-647-1865
Website: www.abct.org

Autism Network International (ANI)

P.O. Box 35448
Syracuse, NY 13235-5448
Website: www.autismnetworkinternational.org

Autism Research Institute (ARI)

4182 Adams Ave.
San Diego, CA 92116
Toll-Free: 833-281-7165
Phone: 619-281-7165
Fax: 619-563-6840
Website: www.autism.org
E-mail: info@autism.org

Autism Science Foundation (ASF)

106 W. 32nd St.
Ste. 182
New York, NY 10001
Phone: 914-810-9100
Website: www.autismsciencefoun-
dation.org
E-mail: contactus@autismscience-
foundation.org

Autism Society of America (ASA)

4340 East-West Hwy
Ste. 350
Bethesda, MD 20814
Toll-Free: 800-328-8476
Website: www.autism-society.org

Depressed Anonymous

P.O. Box 17414
Louisville, KY 40214
Website: www.depressedanon.com
E-mail: depanon@netpenny.net

Depression and Bipolar Support Alliance

55 E. Jackson Blvd.
Chicago, IL 60604
Toll-Free: 800-826-3632
Fax: 312-642-7243
Website: www.dbsalliance.org

Eating Disorder Referral and Information Center

Website: www.edreferral.com

Families for Depression Awareness

391 Totten Pond Rd.
Ste. 101
Waltham, MA 02451
Phone: 781-890-0220
Fax: 781-890-2411
Website: www.familyaware.org
E-mail: info@familyaware.org

Mental Health America (MHA)

500 Montgomery St., Ste. 820
Alexandria, VA 22314
Toll-Free: 800-969-6642
Phone: 703-684-7722
Fax: 703-684-5968
Website: www.nmha.org
E-mail: info@mhanational.org

Mental Health Association of Westchester (MHA)

580 White Plains Rd.
Ste. 510
Tarrytown, NY 10591
Phone: 914-345-0700
Website: www.mhawestchester.org
E-mail: help@mhawestchester.org

National Alliance on Mental Illness (NAMI)

3803 N. Fairfax Dr.
Ste. 100
Arlington, VA 22203
Toll-Free: 800-950-NAMI
(800-950-6264)
Phone: 703-524-7600
TDD: 703-516-7227
Fax: 703-524-9094
Website: www.nami.org
E-mail: info@nami.org

National Association of School Psychologists (NASP)

4340 E.W. Hwy
Ste. 402
Bethesda, MD 20814
Toll-Free: 866-331-NASP
(866-331-6277)
Phone: 301-657-0270
TTY: 301-657-4155
Fax: 301-657-0275
Website: www.nasponline.org
E-mail: webmaster@naspweb.org

National Center for Child Traumatic Stress (NCCTS)

NCCTS—University of California,
Los Angeles
11150 W. Olympic Blvd.
Ste. 650
Los Angeles, CA 90064
Phone: 310-235-2633
Fax: 310-235-2612
Website: www.nctsn.org
E-mail: info@nctsn.org

National Center for Victims of Crime (NCVC)

2000 M St. N.W.
Ste. 480
Washington, DC 20036
Phone: 202-467-8700
Fax: 202-467-8701
Website: victimsofcrime.org
E-mail: webmaster@ncvc.org

National Eating Disorders Association (NEDA)

1500 Bdwy.
Ste. 1101
New York, NY 10036
Toll-Free: 800-931-2237
Phone: 212-575-6200
Fax: 212-575-1650
Website: www.nationaleatingdisor-
ders.org
E-mail: info@
NationalEatingDisorders.org

National Organization for People of Color Against Suicide (NOPCAS)

815 Pershing Dr.
Ste. 355
Silver Spring, MD 20910
Phone: 301-529-4699
Website: www.nopcas.org
E-mail: dbarnes@nopcas.org

National Organization for Victim Assistance (NOVA)

510 King St.
Ste. 424
Alexandria, VA 22314
Toll-Free: 800-879-6682
(800-TRY-NOVA)
Phone: 703-535-6682
Fax: 703-535-5500
Website: www.trynova.org

National Register of Health Service Psychologists (NRHSP)

1200 New York Ave., N.W.
Ste. 800
Washington, DC 20005
Phone: 202-783-7663
Fax: 202-347-0550
Website: www.nationalregister.org
E-mail: support@nationalregister.org

Treatment Advocacy Center

200 N. Glebe Rd.
Ste. 801
Arlington, VA 22203
Phone: 703-294-6001
Fax: 703-294-6010
Website: www.treatmentadvocacy-center.org
E-mail: info@treatmentadvocacy-center.org

INDEX

INDEX

Page numbers followed by 'n' indicate a footnote. Page numbers in *italics* indicate a table or illustration.

Index

Index

Index

F

Index

Index

Index

Index

Index

Index

Index